ALZHEIMER'S DISEASE

Advances in

PREVENTION & TREATMENT

2016 Report

A Special Report
published by the editors of
Focus on Healthy Aging
in conjunction with
Icahn School of Medicine at Mount Sinai
New York, New York

Alzheimer's Disease: Advances in Prevention & Treatment

Consulting Editor: Judith Neugroschl, MD, Assistant Professor, Alzheimer's Disease Research Center,
Department of Psychiatry, Icahn School of Medicine at Mount Sinai

Author: Lynne Christensen
Group Directors, Belvoir Media Group: Diane Muhlfeld, Jay Roland
Creative Director, Belvoir Media Group: Judi Crouse
Editor, Belvoir Media Group: Jay Roland
Illustrations: Stacy Jannis, Rebekah Fredenburg, Marty Bee, Thinkstock

Publisher, Belvoir Media Group: Timothy H. Cole

ISBN: 978-1-879620-77-3

To order additional copies of this report or for customer service questions, please call 877-300-0253,
or write to Health Special Reports, 535 Connecticut Avenue, Norwalk, CT 06854.

NEW FINDINGS

- Women at risk for Alzheimer's disease decline faster than men (Page 11, Box 1-1)

- Type 1 diabetes may increase risk for dementia (Page 22, Box 3-1)

- Prediabetes may boost risk for dementia (Page 23, Box 3-2)

- Sleep apnea linked to earlier cognitive decline (Page 26, Box 3-6)

- More olive oil and nuts may boost mental function (Page 31, Box 4-2)

- Diet for brain health (Page 32, Box 4-3)

- Education, occupation, and school grades may affect later risk for dementia (Page 35, Box 4-4)

- Loneliness linked to faster decline in mental function (Page 37, Box 4-5)

- Physical activity helpful for people with Alzheimer's disease (Page 58, Box 7-2)

- Experimental Alzheimer's drug shows promise (Page 88, Box 11-3)

INTRODUCTION

Many people fear getting Alzheimer's disease, a devastating condition that compromises the ability to remember, think, and take care of oneself. There is no cure and the treatments available today can help with symptoms, but only temporarily. Many experts believe that the greatest hope for truly impacting Alzheimer's disease will involve prevention. As of now, no drug or other therapy has been proven to prevent Alzheimer's disease. But there is hope. Many therapies are under investigation and results should be coming in over the next several years.

The imperative to find a solution could not be greater, because a surge in the older adult population has begun and will continue for the next 20 years. This will be accompanied by an increase in age-related illnesses, including Alzheimer's disease. According to the Centers for Disease Control and Prevention (CDC), Alzheimer's disease is the sixth-leading cause of death in the United States and the fifth-leading cause of death for those age 65 and older.

This report contains information for those concerned about getting Alzheimer's disease and those who have been diagnosed with it, as well as caregivers of people with dementia. It will help you identify the differences between normal memory changes and dementia. It also presents the research on what may put some people at greater risk, and sorts out the often conflicting reports about how to reduce risk. You will learn what is known about Alzheimer's disease, and what research laboratories are discovering. For those caring for a loved one with Alzheimer's disease, there is helpful information about caregiving, as well as some practical advice on legal, financial, and health-care arrangements.

Normal forgetfulness

Growing older doesn't necessarily portend a slow decline into forgetfulness and eventual senility. It is common to experience some change in memory with age, but many people maintain their mental faculties throughout their entire lives. For some people, normal age-related decline accelerates and becomes far more serious, impacting the ability to think, learn, remember, and reason. The cause is dementia, the most common form of which is Alzheimer's disease.

There are many misconceptions about memory, age, and Alzheimer's disease. This report helps sort out what is known about Alzheimer's. It describes the disease process, the physical damage that occurs in the brain, and its effect on memory and other cognitive functions.

Many people complain that their memory isn't as sharp as it used to be. In Chapter 2, "Normal Changes in Memory with Age," we differentiate memory changes that are expected with normal aging from memory changes that may indicate a brain disease such as Alzheimer's.

Risk factors

A good deal of research has been done to try to pinpoint who is at greatest risk for getting Alzheimer's disease. While heredity plays a role in one's risk for Alzheimer's disease, other factors also contribute. Chapter 3, "Who Is at Risk for Alzheimer's Disease?" reviews the latest research on risk factors such as genetics, cholesterol, diabetes, depression, smoking, and obesity.

Addressing these risk factors early in life may improve overall health, including brain health, throughout life. Chapter 4, "Can You Reduce Your Risk for Dementia?" discusses vitamins, diet, and the benefits of mental, social, and physical activity. One message from research is that exercise, mental stimulation, and social interaction may help preserve brain function longer. While we're waiting for scientists to locate just the right chemical compounds to treat this devastating disease, there are positive and active steps everyone can take right now. Stay active, stay socially involved, and stay mentally engaged. Even if those steps don't prevent Alzheimer's disease, your brain may be better off because of them.

Diagnosis and symptoms of Alzheimer's

No one test will prove that a person has Alzheimer's disease. However, a skilled physician can conduct a comprehensive evaluation and make the diagnosis with more than 90 percent accuracy. Chapter 5, "Diagnosis," describes some of the tests doctors use to diagnose dementia, and includes some early-warning signs that should prompt you to get evaluated.

A person with Alzheimer's disease will have increasing difficulty with memory, language, time perception, visual-spatial orientation, and problem-solving ability. Mood and behavior changes will also occur. Chapter 6, "How Alzheimer's Disease Affects Mental Function," describes the changes in cognitive functioning that can be expected at each of the three stages of the disease: mild, moderate, and severe.

Treatment and caregiving

Although there's no drug that will cure Alzheimer's disease, there are medications that may slow the decline of the disease. Chapter 7, "Treatment," reviews the drugs that are FDA-approved for Alzheimer's disease. It also discusses other potential treatments, including antioxidants, herbs, and cognitive rehabilitation.

For caregivers, Chapter 8, "Caring for a Person with Alzheimer's Disease," explains what can be reasonably expected from someone with Alzheimer's, and how to handle challenging behaviors. It also describes care options, including adult day-care services, respite care, in-home care, assisted-living, and nursing home care. Chapter 9, "Handling Caregiver Stress," reminds caregivers not to neglect their own health and well-being while caring for a person with Alzheimer's disease.

Practical advice and hope for the future

Receiving an Alzheimer's diagnosis can be emotionally charged, and practical matters may be neglected. But at some point, early on, it will be necessary to make certain financial and legal arrangements. Chapter 10, "Practical Advice: Legal, Financial, Health Care," reviews the types of decisions that will be necessary, including the documents that will need to be drawn up and the types of professionals to consult.

The last chapter, "The Future of Alzheimer's Research," reviews current research efforts and spotlights future initiatives. Scientists are using newly gained knowledge about the underlying causes of Alzheimer's to devise strategies to try to stop the disease in its tracks.

TABLE OF CONTENTS

TABLE OF CONTENTS

WHAT IS ALZHEIMER'S DISEASE?

Just about everyone experiences some memory lapses as they age. You may misplace your reading glasses, forget the name of someone you just met, or not remember where you parked the car. Most memory slips like this can be overcome with memory tricks or being more organized (such as always putting your glasses in the same place). Normal memory problems related to aging are discussed in Chapter 2.

For some people, problems with memory and thinking become increasingly worse, and seriously affect daily life. When this happens dementia is a likely cause. Alzheimer's disease is the most common of several causes of dementia. A condition called mild cognitive impairment falls between normal forgetfulness and dementia.

Mild cognitive impairment

Some older adults have problems with memory, language, and other mental functions that are more pronounced than normal age-related changes but that don't fulfill the criteria for dementia. This condition is called mild cognitive impairment (MCI). If only memory is affected the condition is called amnestic MCI. But people with MCI may also have problems with other types of mental function, such as language and problem solving. For people with MCI these problems are noticeable but they don't seriously impact day-to-day functioning. When they are tested, people who have MCI remember less of a paragraph they have read or details of a simple drawing they have seen compared to people with normal age-related memory changes.

MCI can be, but is not always, a transitional state between normal aging and Alzheimer's disease. Some people with MCI do not get worse and do not develop dementia, and some may even get better. Researchers are looking for specific characteristics that indicate a person with MCI is on the way to developing dementia.

Dementia

The term dementia refers to a severe decline in mental ability. People with dementia have impairments in the brain that affect memory and other types of mental functioning, such as reasoning, judgment, language, and abstract thinking. These problems seriously interfere with daily life. Unlike with age-related forgetfulness, the memory and thinking problems of dementia make normal daily activities like cleaning, organizing, preparing meals, doing household chores, and handling finances increasingly difficult and ultimately impossible. The ability to engage in day-to-day tasks at home, at work, or in social situations become severely diminished over time.

Different causes of dementia can have slightly varying symptoms. They can also overlap. Many people with dementia have more than one type, which is called mixed dementia.

Alzheimer's disease

Alzheimer's disease, which accounts for about 60 to 80 percent of all cases of dementia in the United States, is well known as a memory-robbing disease. But, like with other forms of dementia, people with Alzheimer's disease also have difficulty with other vital mental functions, like language, judgment, and problem solving. They have changes in personality, mood, activity level, and perceptions of the immediate environment. The changes are subtle at first and become worse over the years. Eventually people with Alzheimer's disease must depend on others to care for them (the changes in mental function are described in greater detail in Chapter 6).

About 5.3 million Americans have Alzheimer's disease, according to the Alzheimer's Association. Women are more likely than men to have the disease. Almost two-thirds of all Americans with Alzheimer's disease are women. This may be due to the fact that women, on average, live longer than men, although new research suggests there may be other reasons.

A recent study found that women with mild cognitive impairment (MCI), which often precedes Alzheimer's disease, have faster decline in mental functioning than men with MCI (see Box 1-1, "Women at risk for Alzheimer's decline faster than men"). The reason for the difference between the sexes is not known.

Alzheimer's disease mostly strikes after age 65, but it can also occur as early as age 30 in people with a rare form of hereditary Alzheimer's disease (see page 19, "Genetically determined Alzheimer's disease"). About five percent of people with Alzheimer's disease have the hereditary form that can occur at a younger age.

Eleven percent of Americans aged 65 and older have Alzheimer's disease, and about one-third of people ages 85 and older have it. Most people who have Alzheimer's disease (81 percent) are age 75 or older.

It's important to realize that many people who live into their 80s and 90s retain their mental faculties. A slow decline into senility is not inevitable. Alzheimer's disease is a distinct disease, causing specific abnormal changes in the brain.

Women at risk for Alzheimer's decline faster than men

More women than men have Alzheimer's disease, and the fact that women tend to live longer has been proposed as the reason. But there may be other factors at work, based on a recent study.

Researchers analyzed data on about 400 men and women in their mid-70s who had mild cognitive impairment (MCI). MCI can be a transitional state between normal mental functioning and Alzheimer's disease. After four to seven years, the researchers found that the rate of mental decline in men was half that of women. The reason for faster decline in women is still not known.

Alzheimer's Association International Conference, July 2015

BOX 1-2

NEURONS

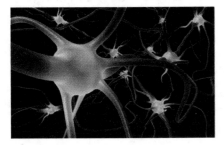

The brain contains about 100 billion neurons.

BOX 1-3

HEALTHY NEURON VS. NEURON WITH ALZHEIMER'S DISEASE

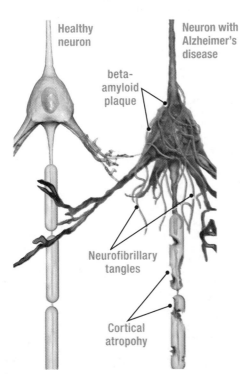

Healthy neuron

Neuron with Alzheimer's disease

beta-amyloid plaque

Neurofibrillary tangles

Cortical atropohy

Although the specific cause of the brain changes in Alzheimer's disease is not known, researchers are working to better understand the mechanisms of the disease.

Other causes of dementia

The second most common type of dementia is vascular dementia. This can occur as a result of damage to blood vessels in the brain that reduces or blocks blood flow. Blocked or diminished blood flow prevents oxygen and vital nutrients from reaching portions of the brain. When major blood vessels are obstructed a stroke can occur, which usually causes obvious symptoms (weakness, numbness of the face, arms, or legs, or trouble speaking). It's also possible to have minor strokes that are barely noticeable at the time (called transient ischemic attacks, or TIAs). The damage from strokes, even a succession of small ones can lead to vascular dementia.

Other causes of dementia are frontotemporal dementia, dementia with Lewy bodies, Huntington's disease, Creutzfeldt-Jakob disease, and normal pressure hydrocephalus. Dementia can also occur in people with Parkinson's disease or alcoholism. Some people have more than ones, form of dementia—for example, a combination of Alzheimer's disease and vascular dementia, or Alzheimer's disease and dementia with Lewy bodies.

Brain changes in Alzheimer's disease

The brain—by far the most complex organ in the body—contains about 100 billion specialized cells called neurons (see Box 1-2, "Neurons"). Neurons are clustered into distinct regions of the brain, each having specialized functions. For example, a region called the hippocampus plays a critical role in memory. The regions of the brain communicate with each other via an extensive two-way network of neurons. This interaction produces all of the functions of the brain, from thoughts, feelings, and memories, to movement and even breathing.

Damage to the brain—from strokes, head injuries, dementia, or other causes—can interfere with normal brain functioning depending on the type of damage and where in the brain it occurs.

Alois Alzheimer, who identified the first Alzheimer's patient in 1906, found two distinctive features when he performed an autopsy on the brain of a patient who had symptoms of dementia before she died. He discovered that nerve cells in certain areas of the brain were gummed up by a sticky material called amyloid plaque. Inside the cells, he found twisted threads called neurofibrillary tangles (see Box 1-3, "Healthy neuron vs. neuron with Alzheimer's disease").

The presence of these plaques and tangles distinguishes Alzheimer's disease from other forms of dementia (see Box 1-4, "Plaques and tangles").

BOX 1-4

Plaques and tangles show up first in the regions of the brain responsible for memory. As the disease progresses, these plaques and tangles rob cells in crucial brain areas of the ability to function. Key brain cells eventually die, which accounts for the permanent problems with memory, thinking, and behavior.

In addition to plaques and tangles, other abnormalities are seen in the brains of people with Alzheimer's disease. These include inflammation and oxidative damage to brain cells (from highly reactive forms of oxygen).

Many questions remain unanswered about the relationship of the plaques and tangles to the disease. For example, do plaques form first, which then cause tangles to form, which leads to the development of Alzheimer's disease? Or, do the tangles occur first? Or, does some other physiologic event happen that triggers the formation of plaques and tangles? These questions have become imperative to answer because researchers now believe that understanding the earliest brain changes is the key to unlocking the mystery of Alzheimer's disease and possibly preventing it.

Amyloid plaques

Amyloid plaques are a sticky byproduct of a substance called beta-amyloid. Beta-amyloid is a small section of a larger protein called amyloid precursor protein (APP), which exists inside neurons. Under normal circumstances, APP appears to aid in the growth and maintenance of neurons. It stimulates the development of nerve paths. Intact nerve paths are essential for the brain to function properly. Through a process not yet fully understood, the APP can get snipped into smaller pieces, like taking a long strand of ribbon and cutting it into smaller sections. Sometimes it gets clipped into harmless pieces and sometimes it gets clipped in such a way that it forms beta-amyloid. Scientists have identified the enzymes that act like scissors, snipping APP into the beta-amyloid fragments.

The short beta-amyloid strands, intermingled with portions of neurons and other cells, clump together and eventually form sticky deposits called plaques. Plaques are found in the spaces between the brain's neurons. In people with Alzheimer's disease, these plaques form first in areas of the brain responsible for memory and thinking. The plaques displace healthy neurons and may kill them. Research is underway to better understand the biological mechanisms of APP, in the hope of discovering a way to stop it from breaking down into the detrimental beta-amyloid.

PLAQUES AND TANGLES

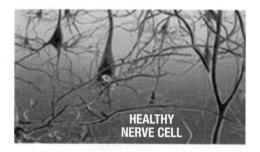

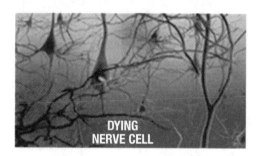

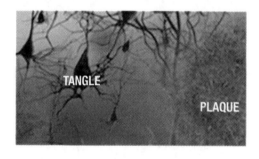

Alzheimer's tissue has far fewer nerve cells and synapses than a healthy brain. Plaques build up between nerve cells. Dead and dying nerve cells contain tangles, which are made up of twisted strands of the protein tau.

Image credit: Jannis Productions. Rebekah Fredenburg, computer animation

BOX 1-5

THE BRAIN AND ALZHEIMER'S DISEASE

Alzheimer's disease attacks nerve cells (neurons) in several areas of the brain, including:

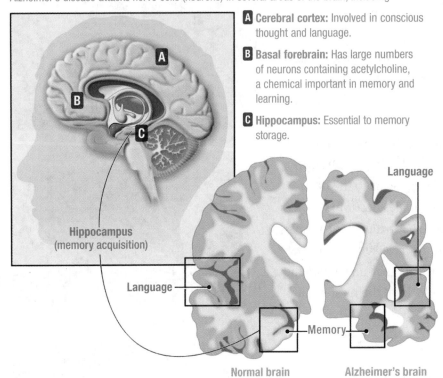

A Cerebral cortex: Involved in conscious thought and language.

B Basal forebrain: Has large numbers of neurons containing acetylcholine, a chemical important in memory and learning.

C Hippocampus: Essential to memory storage.

Hippocampus
(memory acquisition)

Language

Language

Memory

Normal brain   Alzheimer's brain

BOX 1-6

Normal brain vs. Alzheimer's brain

In the Alzheimer's brain the cortex shrivels up, damaging areas involved in thinking, planning and remembering. Shrinkage is especially severe in the hippocampus, an area of the cortex that plays a key role in the formation of new memories. Ventricles (fluid-filled spaces within the brain) grow larger.

Neurofibrillary tangles

Neurofibrillary tangles are dense proteins within neurons that injure the cells. These tangles are twisted threads, the major component of which is a protein called tau. Normally, tau has a beneficial function. But in people with Alzheimer's disease, the tau protein has gone through a chemical change that prevents it from acting normally. The tau threads become twisted up with one another, forming tangles. As a result, the neuron loses the ability to function well, and it ultimately dies.

Lost connections

As plaques and tangles become more numerous, they damage neurons to the point where they can no longer communicate with one another. Neurons communicate via chemicals called neurotransmitters, which carry signals from one cell to another. It is the intricate interconnection of billions of neurons communicating via these signals that regulates all the functions of the brain, from generating thoughts to controlling bodily movements.

Eventually the plaques and tangles cause neurons to die, and vital connections are lost. At first, the loss of neurons primarily affects the parts of the brain responsible for short-term memory (the hippocampus and entorhinal cortex), leading to short-term memory failures (see Box 1-5, "The brain and Alzheimer's disease"). Later, the areas of the brain that control language, attention, and reasoning (in the cerebral cortex) are affected. Damage caused by Alzheimer's disease can spread to other parts of the brain, leading to greater and greater disability. Over time, the brain shrinks dramatically as more and more neurons die (see Box 1-6, "Normal brain vs. Alzheimer's brain").

Scientists don't fully understand the exact sequence of biological events that leads up to Alzheimer's disease, yet there are several hypotheses. It is believed that the plaques, tangles, and other brain changes of Alzheimer's disease begin long before memory loss and other cognitive problems become noticeable. This is discussed in greater detail in Chapter 11.

NORMAL CHANGES IN MEMORY WITH AGE

Many people in middle and older age complain that their memory just isn't as sharp as when they were young. It becomes harder to remember names of people you just met. You may spend more time than you'd like looking around for your reading glasses, watch, or car keys. How many times have you walked into a room only to forget why you went there? As we age memory starts to falter in mostly predictable ways. Increasing difficulty with short-term memory (like forgetting where you parked the car), diminished ability to quickly switch mental gears among several tasks, and taking longer to process new information are typical in most people as they get older.

These problems are not uncommon, and they are not telltale symptoms of dementia. In dementia, cognitive abilities are lost to the point where a person cannot function independently. In normal aging, they are simply diminished somewhat.

Some memory problems may be caused by a health condition or medication you're taking. Fatigue, stress, depression, and anxiety can lower your memory potential, as can a vitamin B12 deficiency, thyroid problems, and anemia. Medications such as antihistamines, anti-anxiety drugs, sleep aids, and painkillers also may impair memory. You can correct the problem by treating the underlying condition or by stopping the medication. Any concerns about medications and their potential cognitive effects or interactions should be discussed with your doctor. Concerning drug interactions, your pharmacist may be a valuable resource of information to bring to your doctors.

Normal memory changes

The changes that take place in memory and cognition vary from person to person; however, some are relatively common. For example, the speed at which the brain processes information is often affected. This means if a list of words is given to a group of 20-year-olds and a group of 75-year-olds, and they are asked to recall the words a short time later, the 20-year-olds will remember more words. However, if the list of words is shown more than once and the participants are allowed to read the words out loud, the 75-year-olds are likely to do just as well as the 20-year-olds. The more exposure you have to information you need to remember, and the more often you repeat it, the more likely you are to remember it, at any age. Therefore, it's possible to compensate for reduced information-processing speed.

Older adults may also experience a delay in recalling information. This is what is happening when you have to rack your brain to remember a familiar word or the name of someone you recently met. The encouraging news is the information is not gone for good. If someone tells you the word or name, you will recognize it, or you may eventually come up with it on your own.

Focus on one task at a time

Some older adults have a decreased ability to divide their attention among more than one activity or source of information. This also happens to people with Alzheimer's disease. With Alzheimer's disease it becomes increasingly worse, significantly impairing the ability to function. With normal aging, it simply means that you need to concentrate your attention more fully on one task at a time.

On the positive side, aging does not affect the recall of established skills. Vocabulary and general knowledge continue to increase with age, and reasoning and intelligence are not impaired.

It is important to realize there are large differences in mental function among people at any age. Not everyone experiences difficulties in all aspects of mental function, and the degree of difficulty varies widely among different people. Some people in their 70s and 80s have a remarkable ability to maintain a very high level of memory and other mental functioning.

The adaptable brain

In the past, age-related changes were blamed on dying neurons in the brain. Experts believed that new neurons were produced only early in life and once a person reached adulthood brain cells started to die off. A much more complex view of the brain has come to be accepted. Neurons don't die quite as rapidly as previously thought and new neurons actually can grow, even in adults.

Perhaps more importantly, new connections among neurons continue to be formed throughout life. Brain processes, including memory, thinking, and other functions, occur as neurons communicate with one another via projections (called axons and dendrites) that create a vast web inside the brain. As memories are formed, new skills learned, or other thought processes occur, new pathways get created among the network of neurons. The more the information is reinforced, the stronger the pathway becomes. Because the brain responds to stimulation, such as exposure to new information, by creating new connections staying mentally active by reading, doing crossword puzzles, joining discussion groups, or engaging in any activity that stretches your mind may help you maintain mental function.

The brain also is capable of adapting. In fact, the brain has a remarkable capacity for modification and repair. If one network becomes faulty, another network can often take over its function. And even if new neurons are not created the existing ones can create new connections.

Memory training

Because the brain is adaptable and can continue to form new connections throughout life, most people can learn and improve their memory at any age. A memory-improvement industry has grown up around the promise of mental fitness. Numerous books and computer- and Web-based products claim to boost memory and mental function. Whether these brain-training programs have any measurable impact on memory or cognition is not known.

Before spending money on a high-tech solution, however, consider some low-tech strategies for improving your memory. Put simply, memory involves three basic steps: acquiring information, storing it, and retrieving it. Often people have difficulty remembering something because they didn't adequately acquire the information to begin with. Acquiring information requires you to focus your attention on what you want to remember. So when you park your car in a large parking lot, stop and be mindful for a moment, telling yourself exactly where your car is and perhaps write down the location—then it will be easier for you to find your car later.

It's easier to pay attention to, and therefore to remember, information that has meaning to you. You can also give meaning to information you find not quite as interesting, making it easier to remember. You can organize the information in certain ways, or use memory tricks. An example of a memory trick is the method commonly used to remember how many days are in each month ("Thirty days hath September, April, June and November…").

Another way to improve your memory is simply to be more organized. Use tools such as appointment books and calendars to keep track of your schedule. Keep a to-do list to remember tasks and chores. Designate certain "forget-me-not spots" where you always put your keys or glasses. Remember, it isn't always necessary to rely on your memory. Keep a notebook in which you write things you want to remember.

You can learn memory techniques (see Box 2-1, "Memory techniques"). For example, you can create a story or picture for things you want to remember or say the information out loud. You can also connect new information with something that you already know well.

BOX 2-1

Memory techniques

There are several techniques you can use to give meaning to information so that you can more easily remember it. Different people prefer different ways of remembering. Choose a method that works for you and keep practicing it. Here are seven techniques for one of the most common memory complaints: recalling names.

1 REPETITION
If you want to learn someone's name, simply repeat it until you've learned it. Say the name silently to yourself or aloud during a conversation, or, if you're on the telephone, write it down while speaking.

2 PRACTICE
This is similar to the repetition method, but it uses a specific structure for the repetition. For example, spell the name (to yourself or out loud), make a remark about the name, or say the person's name at the beginning or end of the conversation.

3 CONNECTION
Make a connection between the name and something that is familiar to you. For example, if the person's name is Noah, say or think, "Oh, as in the ark?" This makes the name more meaningful and memorable.

4 SNAPSHOT
You may not be aware of the strength of your visual memory. Use it by picturing the person's name, which can make abstract information more tangible and meaningful. Some names are easy to visualize (e.g., Green, Shepard, Fox).

5 STORYTELLING
Make a name more meaningful by creating a funny or exaggerated association for it. For example, take the name "Frank Hill." You may say to yourself, "Frankly, he's getting over the hill."

6 MOVIE
This technique uses both verbal and visual associations and involves motion. If you want to remember Earl Brickman, you could picture an earl, dressed in robes, laying bricks.

7 VISUAL LINK
In this technique, you link something about the person's physical appearance to his or her name. So, if you meet Alfred Turnball and you notice that he has a very round chin, you can imagine his chin as a ball turning.

Source: *Total Memory Workout: 8 Steps to Maximum Memory Fitness,* by Cynthia R. Green, Ph.D., Bantam Books, September 1999

WHO IS AT RISK FOR ALZHEIMER'S DISEASE?

Simply getting older raises your risk for Alzheimer's disease, but age alone does not mean a slow decline toward dementia. Beyond age, there are certain factors that may further increase risk. Most likely, several factors interact to set off the chain of events that cause Alzheimer's disease and the process likely begins at a younger age than previously thought. This highlights the need to start taking actions to reduce risk early in life.

Certain risk factors for Alzheimer's disease cannot be altered, such as age and genetics. Other risk factors relate to medical conditions, such as diabetes, cholesterol levels, and depression. Several other potential risk factors have been studied, some of which may play a role.

Risk factors that cannot be changed

Age

The most important risk factor for Alzheimer's disease is advancing age. While simply getting older doesn't cause the disease, the risk for Alzheimer's disease steadily rises over time beyond the 60s. People over age 85, the fastest growing demographic in the United States, are at the highest risk.

Genetics

If a parent, brother, or sister had Alzheimer's disease, does this mean you should worry that you might get it too? This is not an easy question to answer because of the complex genetic basis of the disease. If a parent or sibling had Alzheimer's disease your chances of also getting the disease are higher. This is because you may have inherited genes that make you more susceptible to the disease. In rare cases, people inherit genes that don't just make the disease more likely, they ensure that the person will get it. This genetically determined Alzheimer's disease accounts for just one percent of all people with the disease.

Genetically determined Alzheimer's disease

In people with genetically determined Alzheimer's disease, defects exist in one or more of three genes. People with even one of these genetic defects will develop Alzheimer's disease (usually between ages

30 and 60), and they have a 50 percent chance of passing the gene mutation on to their children.

One of the defective genes causes the production of an abnormal amyloid precursor protein (APP). The APP protein breaks down into a destructive amyloid protein, beta-amyloid. As explained in Chapter 1, amyloid protein forms plaques in the brain, and may be the trigger event of Alzheimer's disease. The two other genes that, when they have mutations, have been connected to early-onset Alzheimer's disease produce proteins called presenilin 1 and presenilin 2. These proteins appear to be involved in the breakdown of APP into beta-amyloid.

Another apparent direct genetic link to Alzheimer's disease occurs in people with Down syndrome, who have three copies of chromosome 21. The APP gene is located on chromosome 21. Due to cognitive impairment caused by Down syndrome, it can be difficult to evaluate these patients for Alzheimer's disease. However, autopsy studies show that the brains of people with Down syndrome all have the plaques and tangles of Alzheimer's disease as they age. Despite the presence of these physical manifestations of Alzheimer's disease, the age of onset of cognitive decline varies, and not all adults with Down syndrome develop dementia.

Genes that increase risk

For most people with Alzheimer's disease no one specific gene caused it. However, genetics probably does play some role. Research has shown that people with a parent, brother, or sister with Alzheimer's are more likely to get the disease. People with two affected parents appear to have an even greater risk.

One likely genetic culprit appears to be a gene that codes for a protein called apolipoprotein E, which has different subtypes (alleles), called E2, E3, and E4. Everyone inherits two of these subtypes, one from each parent. Having the apolipoprotein E4 (ApoE4) allele increases the risk for Alzheimer's disease. But this is where the situation becomes complicated. Simply having a gene for ApoE4 does not necessarily translate into having Alzheimer's disease. Rather, it makes a person more susceptible than someone without the allele.

Some research shows that another apolipoprotein E allele, ApoE2, may actually decrease the risk for Alzheimer's disease. About 10 to 20 percent of people in the United States have one or two copies of ApoE2. ApoE3 is the most common form, and it appears to have no impact on the development of Alzheimer's disease.

ApoE4

Apolipoprotein E is a protein involved in the breakdown of lipids (fats) in the body, and it plays a role in heart disease. It is not clear what role it plays in the development of Alzheimer's disease. However, about 46 percent of people with Alzheimer's disease carry the ApoE4 gene, while it is present in just 14 percent of the general population. People with two genes for ApoE4 (one from each parent) are at greatest risk for the disease, but even people with only one gene for ApoE4 (from only one parent) have an increased risk. One study found that women who carry the ApoE4 gene may be more likely to develop Alzheimer's disease than men who carry the gene.

It is possible to get tested for the presence of ApoE4. However, the test is not recommended because many people who carry the ApoE4 gene will never develop Alzheimer's disease, and some who do not have this risk factor will develop the disease.

Scientists have identified several other genes, in addition to ApoE4, that appear to increase the risk for Alzheimer's disease. A few genes have been discovered that protect against the disease. It is hoped that by identifying these genes researchers can gain insight into the causes of Alzheimer's disease and possibly use that knowledge to develop more effective treatments.

Race

Several studies have examined whether race and ethnicity play any role in risk for Alzheimer's disease. While findings differ among studies, it appears that African-Americans are about twice as likely as whites to develop Alzheimer's disease. Hispanics have about one-and-a-half times the risk. There are several possible reasons for the differences. For example, conditions such as diabetes and high blood pressure, which may increase risk for Alzheimer's disease, are more common in African-Americans and Hispanics than in whites.

Other factors that may account for the difference relate to socioeconomic characteristics. Some conditions that have been linked to higher risk for Alzheimer's disease are low level of education, low income, and living in a rural area as a child. In the United States, African-Americans and Hispanics are more likely than whites to have fewer than 12 years of education and to have low income. Why these socioeconomic conditions would be linked to Alzheimer's disease is not completely understood.

There may be other explanations for the disparity among races, but these haven't yet been discovered.

Other possible risk factors

Research over the past several years has consistently found that certain health conditions and other factors (like smoking) increase a person's risk for developing Alzheimer's disease. In particular, some of the same conditions that make a person more susceptible to heart disease also make dementia more likely. The evidence is strongest for diabetes, high cholesterol, depression, and smoking. Other heart disease risk factors, such as high blood pressure and obesity, have been shown in some studies to increase the chances of getting Alzheimer's disease.

Several studies have shown that the risk from these conditions starts rising when they are present in midlife. For example, in one study people in their early 40s who smoked or had high blood pressure, high cholesterol, or diabetes had a 20 to 40 percent increased risk of developing dementia in older age. People with all four risk factors had double the chance of developing dementia. One study found that treating high blood pressure, high cholesterol, and diabetes may lower the risk for Alzheimer's disease.

Further bolstering the evidence for a link between heart disease risk factors and Alzheimer's disease is a study showing that people who had high cholesterol levels and diabetes prior to being diagnosed with Alzheimer's disease experienced a faster decline in mental function once the disease was diagnosed.

In addition to these risk factors, suffering a moderate or severe head injury increases the risk for Alzheimer's disease and other dementias. Some evidence suggests that anemia, a condition in which the number of red blood cells is lower than normal, may also be linked to an increased risk for Alzheimer's disease.

Diabetes

Having diabetes increases the risk for dementia. Studies have found that people with the more common type 2 diabetes are about twice as likely to develop vascular dementia or Alzheimer's disease as people without diabetes. A recent study found that people with type 1 diabetes, which often begins in childhood, also have a greater chance of getting dementia (see Box 3-1, "Type 1 diabetes increases risk for dementia").

Diabetes is a growing problem in the United States and it particularly affects older adults; 11.8 million people over age 65 (26 percent of people in that age group) have diabetes. Most of these people have type 2 diabetes.

Diabetes is a disease in which the body does not produce or does not properly use insulin. Glucose (a sugar used by the body as a source of energy) is one of the end products of food digestion. Insulin (produced in the pancreas) helps the body to absorb glucose into cells. All organs of the body, including the brain, need glucose to function. But insulin and glucose must be maintained in proper balance in the bloodstream.

In people with type 1 diabetes, the body fails to make insulin. The more common form of diabetes, type 2, is often caused by insulin resistance. This means that the body is producing insulin but is resistant to its effects. In both types of diabetes, the result is too much glucose in the blood. This condition, called hyperglycemia, has numerous detrimental effects, including raising the chance for decline in mental function.

Type 2 diabetes does not occur suddenly. Instead, over time the body becomes more and more resistant to insulin. When blood sugar levels reach a particular threshold diabetes is diagnosed. Research shows that people with blood sugar levels that are higher than normal but not high enough to receive a diagnosis of diabetes (called prediabetes) also appear to be at increased risk for Alzheimer's disease and other forms of dementia (see Box 3-2, "Prediabetes may boost risk for dementia).

In addition to having an increased risk for dementia, older adults with diabetes face a higher risk of developing mild cognitive impairment, a condition that can be a precursor to Alzheimer's disease. And having diabetes may increase the chances a person with mild cognitive impairment will develop Alzheimer's disease.

Excess insulin may also be problematic. Some research suggests that both too much glucose and too much insulin in the blood can increase the amount of beta-amyloid (a feature of Alzheimer's disease) in the brain.

Treatment

Treatment for diabetes is aimed at restoring the balance between insulin and glucose. People with type 1 diabetes must take daily insulin shots, while type 2 diabetes is often treated with diet, exercise, oral medications, and sometimes insulin shots. One study showed that people with poorly controlled diabetes—meaning the balance between insulin and glucose is not consistently maintained—are more likely to develop Alzheimer's disease than people with diabetes that is well controlled. Another study found that older adults with type 2 diabetes who have had episodes of severe drops in blood sugar (hypoglycemia) have higher odds of developing dementia.

Prediabetes may boost risk for dementia

People with higher-than-normal blood sugar levels that indicate they may be on the way to developing type 2 diabetes—a condition called prediabetes—performed worse on tests of memory in a recent study and may be at increased risk for Alzheimer's disease.

The study included 150 adults (average age of 60) with normal mental function who had a parent with Alzheimer's disease or the gene that increases risk. They were given cognitive tests, brain imaging tests, and tests to determine insulin resistance.

The researchers found that in individuals with insulin resistance (a precursor to diabetes), less blood sugar was used by areas of the brain susceptible to Alzheimer's disease, including the hippocampus. And low use of sugar in these brain areas was linked to worse performance on memory tests.

JAMA Neurology, July 27, 2015

It's hoped that the effective treatment of diabetes may reduce the risk of Alzheimer's disease. One study found that people with type 2 diabetes who used the diabetes drug metformin had a lower risk of developing dementia than people taking other commonly used diabetes drugs.

Prevention

The insulin resistance that occurs in people with prediabetes and type 2 diabetes is linked to obesity, a poor diet, and sedentary lifestyle. Healthier lifestyles can reduce insulin resistance. In fact, studies have shown that full-blown type 2 diabetes can be prevented in people with prediabetes who lose weight, eat a healthier diet, and increase physical activity.

High cholesterol

High cholesterol is bad for the heart, and it also may harm the brain. Cholesterol is a fat-like substance that is made in the body and also contained in certain foods, like eggs and meat.

Cholesterol comes in more than one form. The "bad" low-density lipoprotein (LDL) cholesterol can build up in the walls of arteries and block blood flow. The "good" high-density lipoprotein (HDL) cholesterol helps clear excess cholesterol from arteries, thus slowing the dangerous build-up that can lead to heart attacks and strokes.

Research has found that higher levels of HDL cholesterol correlate with better mental functioning. HDL levels can be raised by increasing physical activity and eating foods containing monounsaturated fatty acids, such as olive oil.

When it comes to "bad" (LDL) cholesterol, try to keep levels low throughout life. Studies show that having high cholesterol levels in middle age increases risk for Alzheimer's disease later on. Everyone should have their cholesterol levels checked at least every four to six years and more often if levels are high or you have other risk factors for heart disease. A total cholesterol level of less than 200 mg/dL is ideal. Eating a low-fat diet and getting plenty of exercise can help keep cholesterol levels under control. If those measures don't work, drugs are available to lower LDL cholesterol.

Statins

Drugs used to lower the detrimental LDL cholesterol are called statins. Since high LDL cholesterol raises risk for Alzheimer's disease it seems logical that lowering LDL levels with statin drugs would reduce risk. Several studies looking into this have produced conflicting results. Some studies have been optimistic about the ability of statins to stall the onset of Alzheimer's, while others found no protective effect against Alzheimer's disease.

For now, the bottom line appears to be that having high cholesterol is a risk factor for Alzheimer's disease. Lowering levels of LDL cholesterol, while raising levels of HDL cholesterol, is desirable for heart health and likely for brain health, as well. However, it has not been proven that taking statin drugs lowers the risk for Alzheimer's disease.

Obesity

Obesity, a heart disease risk factor, has been shown to increase the risk for developing Alzheimer's disease. Obesity is defined as having a body mass index (BMI) greater than 30 (see Box 3-3, "What is your BMI?"). Numerous BMI calculators are available online, including one from the National Heart, Lung, and Blood Institute (http://www.nhlbi.nih.gov/health/educational/lose_wt/BMI/bmicalc.htm). Studies have shown that obesity in midlife may raise the chances for dementia later in life. In addition, the location of the excess weight in the body may be as important as simply being overweight. One study found that people with a large belly in their 40s have increased risk for developing dementia in their 70s. Even those who were of normal weight but had

BOX 3-3

WHAT IS YOUR BMI?

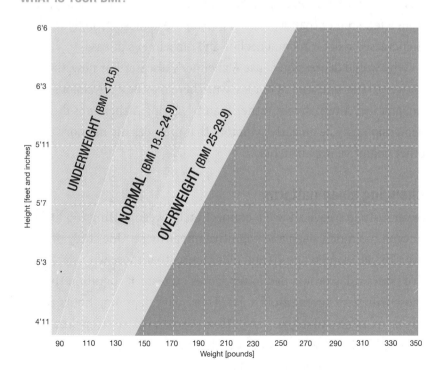

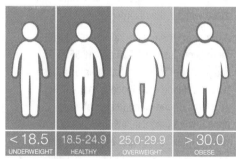

Body mass index (BMI) is one method used to determine obesity. You can estimate your BMI by finding your weight and height in the chart on the left, or you can use the easy online BMI calculators.

A BMI of over 25 is considered overweight, and over 30 is obese.

BOX 3-4

Symptoms of depression

Depression is more than just sadness. Symptoms of depression can include:

- Loss of interest and pleasure in daily activities
- Significant weight loss or gain
- Difficulty sleeping or excessive sleeping
- Lack of energy
- Inability to concentrate
- Feelings of worthlessness or excessive guilt
- Thoughts of death or suicide

Sleep apnea linked to earlier cognitive decline

People with sleep apnea—a disorder that causes gaps in breathing during sleep and usually is accompanied by heavy snoring—may develop mild cognitive impairment (MCI) or Alzheimer's disease at younger ages than those without the disorder.

A group of researchers reviewed medical records of close to 2,500 people 55 to 90 years of age. They found that among those who developed MCI, those with breathing problems during sleep (a sign of sleep apnea) were diagnosed with MCI about 10 years earlier than those with normal sleep patterns—around age 77 compared with around age 90. Among those who developed Alzheimer's disease, it appeared five years earlier in people with disrupted breathing during sleep—age 83 versus age 88.

On a positive note, people with sleep apnea who were treated with a machine that regulates breathing developed MCI 10 years later than those who were not treated—age 82 versus age 72.

Neurology, May 12, 2015

large abdomens were at greater risk than those of normal weight with smaller waists. Obesity plus a large belly resulted in the highest risk, about 3.6 times greater than small-waisted people of normal weight.

One study presents an apparent paradox. It shows that while obesity in middle age increases risk for dementia, after age 65 being underweight has a stronger link to developing dementia than being overweight.

So far, researchers cannot explain the reason for the connection between obesity and dementia. One possibility is the fact that being overweight can lead to high blood pressure, diabetes, and high cholesterol, which all have been shown to contribute to the development of dementia. However, studies have found that being overweight or obese impacts the risk for Alzheimer's disease aside from the presence of diabetes or heart disease. Something about excess body weight appears to trigger damaging brain changes that can lead to dementia.

Depression

About 20 percent of older adults suffer with depression. Signs of this emotional disorder are listed in Box 3-4, "Symptoms of depression." Several studies have concluded that depression increases the risk for developing Alzheimer's disease. However, not all studies have found this link. In addition, there are several unanswered questions, such as whether it matters if depression is major or minor. Also, does it make a difference if depression occurs in early, middle, or late life? It appears from a few studies that depression in later life is most strongly related to increased risk for mental decline and Alzheimer's disease.

Why would depression cause Alzheimer's disease? For now, the answer to this question is not known. There may be a physiologic explanation. Alternatively, rather than triggering Alzheimer's disease, depression may be an early symptom that precedes the memory and other cognitive impairments.

Changing sleep patterns

Several studies have shown a connection between getting too little or even too much sleep and cognitive impairment. One study of over 15,000 women age 70 and older found that those who slept five hours a day or less had lower scores on tests of cognition than those who slept seven hours a day. Those who slept nine hours a day or more also had lower cognition. Women whose sleep duration changed by two hours or more per day had worse cognition than those with no change in sleep duration.

Another study found that participants with sleep apnea or sleep-disordered breathing had more than twice the odds of developing mild cognitive impairment or dementia compared with those without these conditions. In addition, those who woke up more often during the night scored worse on tests of cognition and verbal fluency than those who slept through the night. A more recent study found that mild cognitive impairment and Alzheimer's disease showed up at younger ages in people with sleep apnea, but that treating the disorder might delay the decline in mental function (see Box 3-5, "Sleep apnea linked to earlier cognitive decline.").

The link between poor quality sleep and impaired cognitive function may be causative. In other words, inadequate sleep may lead to dysfunction in the brain that hinders memory and other mental function. But it also may be an early warning sign of dementia. This is not yet known. The connection between sleep and cognitive function continues to be studied.

It is known that getting enough good quality sleep is important for health, including cognitive health, at all ages. In today's busy world, sleep deprivation is all too common. Sleep experts recommend that adults sleep seven to nine hours per night. But the amount of time spent snoozing is declining. On average, we get one to two hours less sleep per night than people did 50 to 100 years ago. An estimated 50 to 70 million Americans have some type of sleep disorder, such as sleep apnea, chronic insomnia, restless legs syndrome, and periodic limb movement disorder.

Sleep specialists recommend "sleep hygiene" techniques to help fall asleep and stay asleep for the recommended seven hours (see Box 3-6, "Sleep hygiene").

Head injury

Some studies have suggested that having a head injury increases the risk for developing Alzheimer's disease. The most common form of head injury is traumatic brain injury (TBI), which can result from a concussion caused by a motor vehicle accident, fall, sports-related injury, or other cause of injury to the head. A TBI can be mild, moderate, or severe. A person with a mild TBI loses consciousness or has loss of memory of the event for less than 30 minutes. If this lasts for more than 30 minutes it is a moderate TBI. With a severe TBI this occurs for more than 24 hours.

Compared with people who have had no head injury, those who experienced a moderate TBI have twice the risk for dementia, and those who had a severe TBI have 4.5 times the risk. The increased

BOX 3-6

Sleep hygiene

The National Sleep Foundation makes several recommendations for getting good quality sleep. These include:

- Maintain a regular sleep and wake cycle. This means going to bed at the same time each night and getting up at the same time each morning.
- Do not nap during the day.
- Avoid caffeine, nicotine, and alcohol close to bedtime.
- Physical activity during the day can help promote sleep. But avoid vigorous exercise close to bedtime.
- Do not eat large meals immediately before bedtime.
- Establish a regular relaxing bedtime routine.
- Make sure your bed is comfortable and your bedroom is quiet, dark, and relaxing. The room should not be too hot or too cold.
- Avoid using your bed for activities other than sleeping and sex, such as watching TV, listening to music, or reading.

risk has not been shown for mild TBI. One study found that older adults with mild cognitive impairment who reported having had a head injury in the past were more likely to have beta-amyloid plaques (a sign of Alzheimer's disease) in their brains than those with no history of head trauma.

Soldiers in combat situations are susceptible to TBIs. In the wars in Afghanistan and Iraq, for example, TBI accounted for 22 percent of all casualties and 59 percent of blast-related injuries. A study of veterans age 55 or older found that those who experienced a previous TBI were 60 percent more likely to develop Alzheimer's disease. In addition, among all veterans in the study who developed dementia, those who had a history of a TBI succumbed to the memory-robbing disorder two years earlier than those who never had a TBI (age 78.5 versus 80.7).

Attention has also been paid to some professional football players diagnosed with dementia at younger ages than would be expected. One study of the cause of death of almost 3,500 NFL players found that death due to neurodegenerative diseases like Alzheimer's disease, Parkinson's disease, and ALS (Lou Gehrig's disease) was three to four times more likely than in the general public. Other studies suggest that cognitive impairment is more prevalent among former professional football players than the general public.

Do these risk factors cause Alzheimer's disease?

It's unlikely that conditions such as high cholesterol, high blood pressure, diabetes, obesity, and smoking directly cause Alzheimer's disease. Rather, they may set the stage for increased vulnerability.

The human body, including the brain, has mechanisms to protect itself from harm. But the detrimental effects of conditions such as high cholesterol may compromise these natural protective mechanisms. For example, the brain needs an adequate amount of blood to flow through its vessels, because blood is the source of the oxygen that nourishes the brain. If these vessels are clogged from the effects of high cholesterol or high blood pressure, the oxygen supply may be reduced, increasing the vulnerability of the brain.

Additionally, high cholesterol, high blood pressure, smoking, and diabetes increase risk for strokes. Many people with Alzheimer's disease actually have mixed dementia, meaning they have both vascular dementia (as a result of prior strokes) and the plaques and tangles of Alzheimer's disease. Perhaps this explains the connection between stroke risk factors and Alzheimer's disease. Or, maybe damage to the brain from strokes makes the brain more susceptible to developing the plaques and tangles of Alzheimer's disease.

Researchers are still trying to untangle the interaction of risk factors and Alzheimer's disease as they search for strategies to intervene early in the course of the disease (even before symptoms are noticed). For example, can disease risk be reduced by lowering blood pressure and cholesterol, and effectively treating diabetes?

The answer is not known. But it appears that keeping cholesterol and blood pressure low, eating a healthy diet, exercising, not smoking and keeping weight under control are good for the heart, as well as for the brain. This is especially important in early adulthood to middle age in order to preserve heart and brain function throughout life.

Cancer and dementia

It appears that having cancer may actually lower risk for Alzheimer's disease. Studies have found that people who've had cancer are less likely to get Alzheimer's disease, and people who have Alzheimer's disease are less likely to develop cancer.

A study that looked at health records of 3.5 million veterans showed that most types of cancer are associated with lower risk for Alzheimer's disease and that chemotherapy treatment for most of the cancers lowered the risk even further. Survivors of liver cancer had the greatest reduction in risk for Alzheimer's disease (51 percent). Other cancers associated with reduced risk were pancreatic cancer (44 percent), esophageal cancer (33 percent), myeloma (26 percent), lung cancer (25 percent), and leukemia (23 percent). Survivors of melanoma and prostate cancer had increased risk. Treatment with chemotherapy reduced Alzheimer's risk by 20 to 45 percent (with the exception of prostate cancer).

So far, researchers cannot explain how cancer and cancer treatment affect brain cells in a way that potentially protects against Alzheimer's disease. There may be other factors not related to cancer at work. Having made this connection, though, may allow researchers to investigate new avenues for potential Alzheimer's treatments.

CAN YOU REDUCE YOUR RISK FOR DEMENTIA?

Unfortunately, no drug exists that has been proven to cure or even prevent Alzheimer's disease or most other forms of dementia. But some evidence suggests that you may be able to lower your risk of developing dementia or at least preserve good mental function longer. Because the disease probably starts long before symptoms appear, it's important to get started early to develop the types of healthy habits that can keep your mind sharp as you age. These relate to diet, exercise and leisure activity.

It's likely that a combination of healthy habits is the key. One study found that a comprehensive program of exercise, social activities, nutritional counseling, and cognitive training, along with management of heart disease risk factors (including high blood pressure and high cholesterol), resulted in better performance on tests of memory and other mental functions.

The evidence is not yet convincing that these actually prevent Alzheimer's. They may help maintain a healthy brain in people without dementia, and many of them (such as eating a low-fat diet and exercising) are good for overall health. A list of steps for maintaining a healthy heart and possibly a healthy brain appears in Box 4-1, "Steps that may reduce your risk for Alzheimer's disease."

BOX 4-1

Steps that may reduce your risk for Alzheimer's disease

Although there is no proven method for preventing Alzheimer's disease, some lifestyle factors may help maintain mental function and possibly lower your risk for dementia:

- Engage in regular physical activity. Physical exercise provides many health benefits, including possibly maintaining and improving cognitive function. Aim for 20 to 30 minutes of aerobic exercise a day on most days.

- Eat a healthy diet with plenty of fruits and vegetables, as well as whole grains and beans (which contain folic acid). Leafy green vegetables contain B vitamins and antioxidants, which may help preserve mental function.

- Keep blood pressure, cholesterol levels, and blood sugar levels under control. Have these numbers checked by a physician, and take steps (through diet, exercise, or medication) to bring them down if necessary.

- Maintain a healthy weight. Because obesity increases risk for Alzheimer's disease, try to keep your weight in the normal range (BMI of 18.5 to 24.9).

- Quit smoking. Smoking has many bad effects on health, including harming brain function.

- Get a good night's sleep. People who get too little sleep or poor quality sleep are more likely to have problems with memory and thinking.

- Engage in mentally stimulating activities. Studies have shown that older adults who stay mentally active by reading, dancing, or playing board games or musical instruments have a reduced risk for dementia.

Food for thought

Several studies have shown that eating a healthy diet might help lower your chances of getting Alzheimer's disease. In particular, foods rich in omega-3 fatty acids (fatty fish, such as tuna and salmon), green, leafy vegetables that are high in B vitamins, and foods containing antioxidants like vitamin E may be beneficial.

Mediterranean diet

Evidence is mounting that adopting a "Mediterranean-style" diet, or something similar, may have some protective effect on mental function. This diet emphasizes fruits, vegetables, whole grains, potatoes, beans, and nuts and seeds. Olive oil is an important source of monounsaturated fat. Dairy products, fish, and poultry are consumed in low to moderate amounts. Little red meat is eaten. Eggs are consumed zero to four times a week. Wine is allowed in low to moderate amounts.

One study of more than 17,000 people found that those who most closely adhered to this type of diet were 19 percent less likely to have impaired mental function. In a recent study people who consumed even more olive oil and nuts than recommended in the standard Mediterranean diet had better memory and thinking abilities than people simply advised to eat a low-fat diet (see Box 4-2, "More olive oil and nuts may boost mental function"). Another group of researchers looked specifically at whether diet might reduce risk for Alzheimer's disease. They used a diet that is a combination of the Mediterranean diet and the heart healthy DASH (Dietary Approaches to Stop Hypertension) diet (see Box 4-3, "Diet for brain health," on the following page).

The key ingredients of these diets may be the vegetables, particularly green, leafy ones. In one study, people who ate at least 2.8 servings of vegetables a day had a 40 percent slower rate of cognitive decline than those who ate less than one serving per day. Eating green, leafy vegetables produced the slowest rate of decline. The reason for the positive effect of vegetables on mental function is not known, but it may be related to the fact that vegetables contain vitamins such as E, B6, and B12.

Yet another study found that people who consumed fruits and vegetables daily had a 30 percent reduction in dementia risk. Eating fish at least once a week was associated with a 40 percent reduction in risk, but only for people who were not carriers of the ApoE4 gene (the Alzheimer's disease susceptibility gene). People who regularly used oils rich in omega-3s (such as canola oil, flaxseed oil, and

---

NEW FINDING BOX 4-2

More olive oil and nuts may boost mental function

The Mediterranean-style diet has components that promote overall health, including plentiful vegetables. But two ingredients of the diet may have particular benefits for brain health: olive oil and nuts.

A group of Spanish researchers studied 447 women without dementia but at high risk for heart disease who were around 67 years old at the beginning of the study. Participants were divided into three groups. One group ate a Mediterranean diet that included 1 liter (about 33 ounces) of olive oil a week. The second group also ate a Mediterranean diet, but with an added 30 grams (about 1 ounce) of mixed nuts a day. The third group was advised to eat a low-fat diet.

After about four years participants in the two Mediterranean diet groups scored higher on tests of mental function than at the beginning of the study. They also had higher scores than those on a low-fat diet.

JAMA Internal Medicine, July 1, 2015

Diet for brain health

Several studies have found that eating a healthy diet seems to help preserve mental function. A group of researchers sought to discover whether this would translate to decreased risk for Alzheimer's disease.

They analyzed food questionnaires filled out by 923 people ages 58 to 98 who were followed for four to five years. Some participants followed a Mediterranean diet and some followed a DASH diet. Others conformed to a diet that is a hybrid of these two diets and called the MIND diet. It emphasizes vegetables, particularly leafy green ones (like kale and spinach), whole grains, beans, poultry, and fish. The diet allows for small amounts of red meat and butter.

The researchers found that study participants who strictly adhered to all three diets had a lower risk for Alzheimer's disease compared to those who did not follow the diets. Those who strictly followed the MIND diet had a 53 percent lower risk and those who only stuck to it moderately well reduced their risk 35 percent.

Alzheimer's & Dementia, February 11, 2015

walnut oil) had a 60 percent lower dementia risk compared with those who did not regularly consume these oils.

Unsaturated fat (from olive oil, vegetable oil, fish, and other sources) seems to be beneficial. One study found that saturated fat, which is present in meat (beef, lamb, pork, poultry) and dairy products (butter, cheese, whole milk) may be detrimental.

Fish as brain food

Evidence showing that omega-3 fatty acids benefit brain function comes from studies in both humans and mice. Omega-3 fatty acids are found in fish such as salmon, tuna, herring, and sardines. Several epidemiologic studies have found a connection between consuming fish one or more times per week and reduced risk of developing Alzheimer's disease, compared to people who rarely or never eat fish.

Studies in mice also show a benefit for omega-3 fatty acids. One study was conducted in specialized laboratory mice that were genetically engineered to develop the brain abnormalities of Alzheimer's disease. Researchers tested the effects of one omega-3 fatty acid, docosahexaenoic acid (DHA). Mice fed a diet high in DHA performed better on a memory test and had less damage to their brains than mice fed a diet deficient in DHA.

A study in humans found that the participants who ate the most fish had lower levels of beta-amyloid 40 and beta-amyloid 42 in their blood.

Alcohol

Red wine may offer some benefit, but be careful not to overdo it. Studies have found that moderate alcohol consumption (mostly in the form of red wine) may have a moderate effect on reducing risk for Alzheimer's disease. The mechanism by which alcohol might protect the brain is not known. Excessive drinking is certainly not recommended because it may increase the risk for damage to the brain. Some studies have found that heavy drinking increases the risk for cognitive impairment. In addition, drinking alcohol while taking certain medications can be harmful.

Do B vitamins help?

It has long been known that a vitamin B12 deficiency can cause a form of dementia that differs from Alzheimer's disease. If caught early and treated with vitamin B12 supplementation, this type of dementia is reversible.

The B vitamins (B6, B12, and folic acid) may also have a role in Alzheimer's disease. This is related to their effect on homocysteine, an amino acid (the building blocks of proteins) that is present in the blood. High levels of homocysteine have been associated with a higher risk for heart disease, stroke, and Alzheimer's disease. The B vitamins help to break down homocysteine, and a lack of these vitamins allows homocysteine to build up in the bloodstream.

For this reason it is important to obtain at least the minimum recommended dietary allowance (RDA) of B vitamins to prevent a deficiency. The importance of these vitamins on mental function is supported by several studies.

Vitamins B6 and B12 are found in animal products, while folic acid is contained in leafy green vegetables, orange juice, and fortified breads and cereals.

Because some older adults don't secrete enough gastric acid to properly absorb vitamin B12 from food, taking a B12 supplement is a safe and simple strategy to ensure that your body is receiving adequate amounts of this important nutrient. Additionally, older adults should consider having an annual blood test as part of a routine physical examination to check for B12 deficiency.

Should you take antioxidants, such as vitamin E?

Antioxidant vitamins (C, E, and beta-carotene) help eliminate free radicals—highly reactive molecules that can damage cells in the brain and elsewhere in the body. Because there is evidence of free radical damage in the brains of Alzheimer's disease patients, it is theorized that these antioxidant vitamins can offer protection against Alzheimer's. In particular, vitamin E has been thought to lower the risk for Alzheimer's disease.

Several studies have looked at whether any of these vitamins protect against Alzheimer's disease, with conflicting findings. One study found that people who obtained high amounts of vitamin E from the food they ate were less likely to develop Alzheimer's disease compared to people who consumed the lowest amounts of vitamin E. The same was not found to be true for the other antioxidant vitamins.

One study found that people who took supplements containing a combination of 400 International Units (IU) of vitamin E and 500 milligrams (mg) of vitamin C had a reduced risk for Alzheimer's disease. Another study looked at the intake of vitamins C, E, and beta-carotene in both food and as supplements. This study found that none of them reduced the risk for Alzheimer's disease.

The National Institute on Aging is conducting a study called the Prevention of Alzheimer's Disease by Vitamin E and Selenium (PREADVISE) trial to examine whether taking vitamin E and/or selenium supplements over a period of seven to 12 years can prevent dementia. This study is not yet completed.

Many common foods contain antioxidants, so eating a well-balanced diet can help ensure that you are getting at least the RDA of these vitamins. Vitamin C is found in citrus fruits, tomatoes, red and green bell peppers, broccoli, strawberries, cabbage, spinach, and collard greens. The RDA of vitamin C is 75 mg per day for women and 90 mg for men.

Vitamin E can be obtained from soybean, corn, cottonseed, and safflower oils. Nuts, seeds, and wheat germ are also good sources, as are leafy green vegetables. The RDA for vitamin E is 22 IU.

Beta-carotene can be found in carrots, sweet potatoes, cantaloupe, and other fruits and vegetables that are a deep red, orange, or yellow color. Some dark-green vegetables, such as broccoli, kale, and spinach, also contain beta-carotene.

The question is, does it make sense to take supplements with quantities of these vitamins (particularly vitamin E) that far surpass the RDA? The answer is not currently known.

Some doctors recommend that their patients take a daily supplement of up to 200 to 400 IU of vitamin E. However, because vitamin E thins the blood, high doses (more than 2,000 IU) can be dangerous. Anyone on medications, particularly the blood-thinning drug warfarin (Coumadin), should consult with their doctor before taking a vitamin E supplement.

In addition, one meta-analysis of a number of studies has found that doses of vitamin E exceeding 400 IU may slightly increase your risk of dying. Although the increased risk was very small, it's best to ask your doctor before routinely taking more than 400 IU of vitamin E per day.

Education and mental stimulation

People with higher levels of education and those with mentally challenging jobs appear to be at lower risk for Alzheimer's disease and other forms of dementia. Many experts believe that education and mental stimulation don't actually prevent dementia. Instead, they confer a benefit to the brain that allows the person to maintain normal mental function longer even as plaques and tangles and other damage are developing in the brain. This is called "cognitive reserve."

People with more education are able to compensate longer for cognitive difficulties than those with less education. Thus, it may be that more highly educated people have a delay in the onset of the most mentally debilitating stage of the disease.

Two recent studies found that education even at a young age may impact later risk for dementia. The researchers looked at the relationship between education (including school grades at age 10) and occupation and development of dementia in older age (see Box 4-4, "Education, occupation, and school grades may affect later risk for dementia").

Education is clearly beneficial. But any mentally stimulating activity may help. One study found that engaging in intellectual activity throughout life, at work and in leisure time activities, may delay the onset of cognitive decline for several years. Interestingly, this study found that despite the level of education or mental stimulation involved in work, engaging in activities that require brain power (reading, playing games, using a computer) in mid- to late-life was beneficial.

One study found that people at risk for Alzheimer's disease (because they were carriers of the ApoE4 gene or had a parent with Alzheimer's disease) who frequently played games and did crossword puzzles performed better on tests of memory and other mental function. Brain scans showed that the game players also had greater volume in brain areas involved in memory (such as the hippocampus).

A study of adults ages 75 to 85, who were followed for 21 years, found that those who participated in leisure activities, such as reading, board games, musical instruments, and dancing, had a 63 percent lower risk of developing dementia. Other studies looking at the effects of activities such as reading, playing board games, knitting, gardening, and dancing have come to a similar conclusion.

Benefits of physical and social activity
Physical activity

Several large, well-designed studies have concluded that exercise is good for the brain. Even moderate exercise, such as walking, when done regularly, has proven benefits for mental function. The evidence is convincing that regular physical activity (walking, bicycling, swimming) improves mental function. A few studies also suggest that it may reduce the risk for Alzheimer's disease.

Here's some of the evidence for improved mental function: A study of 124 previously sedentary adults (ages 60 to 75) compared the effects of aerobic exercise (walking) to anaerobic exercise (stretching) on different aspects of mental function, such as memory and executive

NEW FINDING   BOX 4-4

Education, occupation, and school grades may affect later risk for dementia

Having more years of education has been linked to reduced risk for dementia, or at least delayed onset. Two studies found that the connection between education and dementia risk may actually begin at a young age.

One study from Sweden collected information on school performance, education, and occupational attainment on over 7,500 people age 65 and older, including school grades going back to age 10. Those with the lowest grades in childhood had a 21 percent increased risk for dementia later in life. Those who had occupations that required working with data and numbers had a 23 percent lower risk for dementia. The lowest risk (39 percent reduction) was seen in people who had both high grades in childhood and worked in mentally challenging jobs.

A second Swedish study analyzed data on 440 men and women age 75 and older who did not have dementia at the beginning of the study. After nine years, 163 of them developed dementia. The risk for dementia was 50 percent higher for those with the lowest grades when they were 9 or 10 years old. Women whose occupations were complex and required them to work with people (negotiating, instructing, or supervising) had a 60 percent reduced risk for dementia.

Alzheimer's Association International Conference, July 2015

processes (such as planning and scheduling). Participants who engaged in a regular aerobic exercise program showed significant improvement in performing mental tasks, while those in the other group did not.

The Nurses' Health Study has been collecting data on thousands of female nurses for more than three decades. In part of this study, researchers analyzed data on more than 18,000 women, ages 70 to 81, to determine how physical activity affects mental function. Women who were the most physically active scored highest on tests of mental performance; they had a 20 percent lower risk of mental impairment than women who were the least active. In this study, physical activity did not have to be strenuous. Women who walked at a leisurely pace for at least six hours per week had improved mental function. Even women who walked for just two to three hours per week did better on tests of cognition than sedentary women.

Studies in men have produced similar findings. In the Honolulu-Asia Aging Study, researchers looked at the relationship of physical activity (specifically walking) to dementia in 2,257 men, ages 71 to 93. Men who walked less than one-quarter mile each day had almost twice the risk of developing dementia as men who walked more than two miles each day.

Some evidence shows that regular exercise may do more than improve current mental function. It may prevent or at least delay the onset of Alzheimer's disease or mild cognitive impairment. One study found that people who have the ApoE4 gene (which increases risk for Alzheimer's disease) and engage in regular physical activity had no shrinkage in the hippocampus (a brain region responsible for memory that is affected by Alzheimer's disease) compared with a three percent smaller size of that brain region in their sedentary counterparts.

Another study found that physical exercise in middle age and later in life may decrease risk for mild cognitive impairment—a condition that can lead to dementia in some people.

Physical activity has been shown to lower risk for stroke, heart disease, and diabetes, all of which can have a detrimental effect on memory. Preventing these conditions may also help to stave off dementia.

You don't have to become a marathon runner to achieve the benefits, but some form of regular physical activity is important. Try to get 20 to 30 minutes of moderate-intensity exercise on most days. This can be a brisk walk or some other type of exercise that you enjoy. Even greater health benefits can be gained from more vigorous activity for longer periods of time.

Social support

Exercise is clearly good for you, but walking with a friend may be even better. In a Swedish study of 800 men and women age 75 and older, researchers found that leisure activities combining social, mental, and physical activity helped protect mental functioning over the long term. Those who engaged in the most mental, physical, and social activities had a lower risk for developing dementia, and the greatest effect was among people who engaged in all such activities.

Maintaining an active social life has been touted by several researchers as being beneficial to the brain. One study found that people who are both socially active and not easily stressed have a lower likelihood of developing dementia. Loneliness may have the opposite effect. One recent study found that being lonely may accelerate decline in memory and thinking (see Box 4-5, "Loneliness linked to faster decline in mental function"). And having a greater purpose in life was found to reduce the risk for Alzheimer's disease.

Keep in mind

Some caveats regarding research on physical, mental, and social activity must be noted. For example, cause-and-effect relationships between mental or physical exercise and reduced risk for Alzheimer's disease are very difficult to prove. It may be that people who do not suffer from dementia are simply better able to engage in more complex mental tasks. People who later develop dementia may have a less-active social life because they are experiencing subtle early symptoms of the disease. And people with Alzheimer's disease may simply exercise less than those without dementia. The early and subtle manifestations of the disease could impair a person's motivation or ability to organize and follow through with an exercise plan.

It is possible that the difference in rates of Alzheimer's disease between highly educated and less-educated people is actually linked to socioeconomic status. Less-educated individuals are likely to be in a lower socioeconomic group and have less access to medical care. Without adequate health care, they are more likely to have untreated high blood pressure, diabetes, and other conditions that have been shown to increase risk for Alzheimer's disease.

No physical, mental, or social activity can guarantee protection against Alzheimer's disease. Even people who stay intellectually engaged and physically active into older age can succumb to the disease. On the other hand, there's no harm in reading books, doing crossword puzzles, dancing, walking, visiting friends, and engaging in hobbies.

DIAGNOSIS

Alzheimer's disease actually starts to develop before symptoms become apparent. The plaques and tangles most likely exist within the brain for years, until they eventually cause enough damage for changes in memory and mental function to become noticeable. Because the brain begins changing before behavior does, it's important to look for signs of the disease early. Some drugs are effective in improving mental function in the mild-to-moderate stages of the disease. However, early detection can be difficult because the onset of the disease is usually subtle, and the cognitive changes can vary from person to person.

Early warning signs

Many people fear that everyday acts of forgetfulness, such as not remembering where you put your car keys, are early signs of Alzheimer's disease. Although forgetfulness can be an early warning sign of Alzheimer's, the memory loss of Alzheimer's disease is more serious than normal age-related memory difficulties. Misplacing your keys only to find them later is not uncommon. Placing the keys in an odd or inappropriate location, such as inside the sugar bowl, and completely forgetting about it indicates a more serious problem.

With Alzheimer's disease, forgetfulness is a consistent problem, and the information generally is not recalled later, as it often is with normal aging. Also, Alzheimer's disease affects more than just memory. Language, behavior, and the ability to handle day-to-day tasks also become compromised.

To help recognize the warning signs of Alzheimer's disease, and to distinguish them from normal memory lapses, the Alzheimer's Association has developed a checklist of common symptoms. These are listed in Box 5-1, "10 warning signs of Alzheimer's disease."

Alzheimer's disease begins with mild symptoms and gets worse over time. For most people, memory problems will surface first. Difficulty with other cognitive functions, such as language and judgment, will also occur. Some people are aware of the cognitive decline, while others are not. In many cases, relatives and friends first notice a problem. If you suspect that you or a loved one has cognitive impairment, see a physician. A primary care physician may refer you to a neurologist or psychiatrist for evaluation. You also may see a neuropsychologist for additional tests.

BOX 5-1

10 warning signs of Alzheimer's disease

If you recognize several of these symptoms in yourself or a loved one, consult a physician who can properly diagnose the condition.

1 **Memory loss that disrupts daily life.** One of the most common signs of Alzheimer's is forgetting recently learned information. Others include forgetting important dates or events; asking for the same information over and over; relying on memory aides (e.g., reminder notes or electronic devices) or family members for things they used to handle on their own. What's normal? Sometimes forgetting names or appointments, but remembering them later.

2 **Challenges in planning or solving problems.** Some people may experience changes in their ability to develop and follow a plan or work with numbers. They may have trouble following a familiar recipe or keeping track of monthly bills. They may have difficulty concentrating and take much longer to do things than they did before. What's normal? Making occasional errors when balancing a checkbook.

3 **Difficulty completing familiar tasks at home, at work or at leisure.** People with Alzheimer's often find it hard to complete daily tasks. Sometimes, people may have trouble driving to a familiar location, managing a budget at work or remembering the rules of a favorite game. What's normal? Occasionally needing help to use the settings on a microwave or to record a television show.

4 **Confusion with time or place.** People with Alzheimer's can lose track of dates, seasons and the passage of time. They may have trouble understanding something if it is not happening immediately. Sometimes they may forget where they are or how they got there. What's normal? Getting confused about the day of the week but figuring it out later.

5 **Trouble understanding visual images and spatial relationships.** For some people, having vision problems is a sign of Alzheimer's. They may have difficulty reading, judging distance, and determining color or contrast. In terms of perception, they may pass a mirror and think someone else is in the room. They may not realize they are the person in the mirror. What's normal? Vision changes related to cataracts.

6 **New problems with words in speaking or writing.** People with Alzheimer's may have trouble following or joining a conversation. They may stop in the middle of a conversation and have no idea how to continue or they may repeat themselves. They may struggle with vocabulary, have problems finding the right word, or call things by the wrong name (e.g., calling a "watch" a "hand-clock"). What's normal? Sometimes having trouble finding the right word.

7 **Misplacing things and losing the ability to retrace steps.** A person with Alzheimer's disease may put things in unusual places. They may lose things and be unable to go back over their steps to find them again. Sometimes, they may accuse others of stealing. This may occur more frequently over time. What's normal? Misplacing things from time to time, such as a pair of glasses or the remote control.

8 **Decreased or poor judgment.** People with Alzheimer's may experience changes in judgment or decision-making. For example, they may use poor judgment when dealing with money, giving large amounts to telemarketers. They may pay less attention to grooming or keeping themselves clean. What's normal? Making a bad decision once in a while.

9 **Withdrawal from work or social activities.** People with Alzheimer's may start to remove themselves from hobbies, social activities, work projects, or sports. They may have trouble keeping up with a favorite sports team or remembering how to complete a favorite hobby. They may also avoid being social because of the changes they have experienced. What's normal? Sometimes feeling weary of work, family, and social obligations.

10 **Changes in mood and personality.** The moods and personalities of people with Alzheimer's can change. They can become confused, suspicious, depressed, fearful, or anxious. They may be easily upset at home, at work, with friends, or in places where they are out of their comfort zone. What's normal? Developing very specific ways of doing things and becoming irritable when a routine is disrupted.

Source: The Alzheimer's Association

Diagnostic evaluation

No single comprehensive diagnostic test detects Alzheimer's disease. Researchers are making great progress in developing new techniques that can potentially allow physicians to diagnose Alzheimer's disease at an early stage, but many of these technologies are not ready for routine use.

With tests available today it is almost always possible to diagnose dementia. It may be more difficult to identify the type of dementia. Therefore, a thorough diagnostic examination is important because other problems, aside from Alzheimer's disease, may cause dementia. Other possible causes of dementia include stroke, vitamin B12 deficiency, hypothyroidism, normal pressure hydrocephalus (NPH), certain medications, Parkinson's disease, depression, and other illnesses (see Box 5-2, "Causes of dementia").

With some of these conditions, such as B12 deficiency, hypothyroidism, and NPH, dementia is reversible with early treatment. If a medication is causing the problem, stopping the drug or changing the dosage often will correct the cognitive impairment.

The first step in the diagnostic evaluation is to conduct a thorough medical history, followed by physical, psychological, and neurological exams. Blood will be drawn to test for thyroid function and vitamin levels (specifically vitamin B12 and folate).

Brain imaging

Brain imaging studies will most likely be included. The most common methods of imaging the brain are the computed tomography (CT) scan and magnetic resonance imaging (MRI). Although certain findings on these scans may support a diagnosis of Alzheimer's disease, their primary purpose is to look for evidence of tumors, severe head trauma, or prior strokes. The detection of prior strokes doesn't completely rule out Alzheimer's disease because these two forms of dementia can coexist. But it's important to know whether strokes have caused cognitive impairment so you can take steps to prevent future strokes.

A CT scan also can help to distinguish NPH from Alzheimer's disease. In NPH, an abnormal accumulation of fluid surrounding the brain and spinal cord can cause cognitive impairment, gait problems, and urinary incontinence, all of which also may be features of Alzheimer's disease, although in Alzheimer's these are usually not the initial symptoms. The fluid accumulation can be seen on a CT scan. NPH is treated by draining the fluid, which reverses the symptoms in many people.

Tests of mental function

Important diagnostic information is further gleaned from tests of cognitive ability. These range from brief screening tests—often given by a doctor during the initial visit—to in-depth evaluations performed by a neuropsychologist. One commonly used short test is called the Mini-Mental State Examination (MMSE), which is a series of questions that evaluate a person's orientation, attention, language, and calculation ability (see Box 5-3, "Test of cognitive ability: Mini-Mental State Examination [MMSE]"). This test, which can be performed in

BOX 5-3

Test of cognitive ability: Mini-mental state examination [MMSE]

The MMSE is often used in an initial interview with a doctor when dementia is suspected. Here are the questions it asks:

ORIENTATION

- What is the date: (year) (season) (day) (month)?
- Where are we: (state) (county) (town) (hospital) (floor)?

REGISTRATION

- Name three unrelated objects. Allow one second to say each.
- Repeat all three after the test administrator has said them. Repeat them until you learn all three objects.
- Get one point for each correct answer.

ATTENTION AND CALCULATION

- Count backward from 100 by sevens. Stop after five.
- Get one point for each correct answer.

RECALL

- Recall the three objects previously stated.
- Get one point for each correct answer.

LANGUAGE

- Look at a wristwatch and tell the test administrator what it is.
- Repeat for pencil.

REPEAT THE FOLLOWING: "NO IFS, ANDS, OR BUTS."

FOLLOW A THREE-STAGE COMMAND:

1. "Take a paper in your right hand, fold it in half, and put it on the floor."
2. Read and obey the following sentence, which has been written on a piece of paper: "Close your eyes."
3. Write a sentence.

COPY THE ILLUSTRATION TO THE RIGHT.

- All 10 angles must be present and two must intersect.

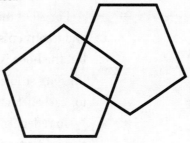

about eight minutes, is helpful, but it has some limitations. Patients with mild-stage Alzheimer's disease who are highly educated may get a perfect score, while people with minimal education or who are not questioned in their primary language may get a low score even though they don't have dementia.

Another simple test that some physicians use to determine if someone should have a more thorough evaluation is the Montreal Cognitive Assessment (MoCA). This test takes about 12 minutes and includes assessment of some mental functions that are not part of the MMSE.

If the quick screening tests done by a physician show problems with memory and thinking, more comprehensive tests of cognitive ability will be performed by a trained professional, such as a neuropsychologist.

Making the diagnosis

Once all other forms of dementia have been ruled out, a doctor will make a diagnosis of "probable" Alzheimer's disease. At this point, the patient and family need to consider appropriate care plans, safety measures, and treatment options.

This is also a good time to join a support group or to otherwise seek help with the psychological impact of receiving the diagnosis. A physician can make the diagnosis, but he or she may not have the resources to help the patient and family cope with the situation they now face. Support groups are available for both people with Alzheimer's disease and their caregivers. The Alzheimer's Association is a good source for finding these groups (see *Resources*, page 96).

Diagnostic criteria

For many years Alzheimer's disease was considered to begin around the time a diagnosis was made using the methods described above. However, it is known that the disease process actually begins before the diagnosis can be made. Researchers now believe that effective treatments for Alzheimer's disease will most likely be effective only if given very early in the course of the disease.

For all of the pieces to come together, the diagnosis must be made and treatments given before symptoms appear. This is not yet possible, but the hope is that it will be in the near future. New tests that use imaging studies and blood and other tests have shown great promise for early detection. These are described in greater detail in Chapter 11.

To reflect the deeper understanding of Alzheimer's disease and to prepare for future advancements in diagnosis and treatment, the

National Institute on Aging and the Alzheimer's Association revised the diagnostic guidelines. The updated guidelines cover the full spectrum of the disease as it gradually changes over many years. They describe three distinct stages of Alzheimer's disease: the earliest preclinical stage (before symptoms appear), mild cognitive impairment (MCI), and dementia due to Alzheimer's disease.

1. Preclinical

In this stage, brain changes have begun but symptoms are not evident. In some people, buildup of beta amyloid in the brain can be detected with new, experimental tests. These are used only in research settings. Currently, this stage is used only in the context of a research study, and the diagnostic parameters are still being evaluated.

2. MCI

The MCI stage is marked by symptoms of memory problems, enough to be noticed and measured, but not compromising a person's independence. People with MCI may or may not develop Alzheimer's dementia. For now, the guidelines for the MCI stage are also largely for research purposes.

3. Alzheimer's dementia

These criteria apply to the stage of the disease when symptoms are evident and causing problems.

HOW ALZHEIMER'S DISEASE AFFECTS MENTAL FUNCTION

The diagnostic criteria refer to three stages of Alzheimer's and include a preclinical stage and mild cognitive impairment (MCI) as the first two stages. Alzheimer's symptoms cause functional impairment in the third stage. This stage is further divided into mild, moderate, and severe. In the mild stage of Alzheimer's disease the symptoms may not be obvious. Day-to-day activities may be only minimally affected. As brain cells continue to die and connections between nerve cells are lost, the symptoms increase and worsen. Because the disease affects people differently, not everyone will lose function in the exact same way. However, for most people, memory loss is the first noticeable sign of Alzheimer's disease.

Changes in memory

Early in the course of the illness, a person with Alzheimer's disease will tend to forget recent events and new information, while retaining memories of past events. Forgetting recent events may cause the person to ask the same questions repeatedly. Eventually, the person may not remember the names or identities of family members or close friends, and long-term memory will be lost as well. This memory loss causes the patient to have difficulty learning new information.

Memory is not one simple function, but a collection of several memory systems. For example, remembering how to drive a car involves a different memory system from that used to remember your wedding day, or from the one that allows you to do mental calculations.

With Alzheimer's disease, recollection of facts and events (called "declarative" memory) tends to become impaired first, particularly with recently acquired memories. With this disruption, it's easy to forget appointments and the content of conversations. A person with Alzheimer's disease may ask a question, get an answer, and then ask the same question five minutes later. Often, people in the mild stage of Alzheimer's disease will be confused about recent experiences, although they have excellent recall of events that occurred 20 years ago. It may be easier to define vocabulary words than to supply recent autobiographical details (such as what the person did yesterday).

Memories of previously acquired skills and procedures, such as playing golf or mowing the lawn (called "procedural" memory), remain intact longer. These well-learned routines hold up for a while, and it may be possible to learn new routines that make use of the procedural memory system.

Alzheimer's disease damages another system called "working memory." Working memory allows you to mentally hold onto information while processing it. For example, arithmetic is performed in working memory. A person with Alzheimer's disease may be able to remember a string of numbers for a short time, but be unable to add or subtract them. Working memory also helps us divide our attention. A person with normal memory can participate in a conversation while remembering that he has to turn off the oven in five minutes. A person with Alzheimer's disease has increasing difficulty dividing his attention, so the oven stays on.

In general, in the mild stage of Alzheimer's disease, it's more difficult to learn new information, and people are more likely to forget recent events than events that occurred in the past. As a result, it becomes increasingly more difficult to perform daily activities, such as shopping, cooking, or keeping appointments.

In the moderate stage of the disease, the memory loss worsens, but highly learned information (such as the person's birthday) and procedural memory (how to brush the teeth) are usually retained. In this stage, the names and identities of family members or close friends may become confused.

In the severe stage, long-term memories will gradually fade, along with highly learned information and activities. The person may still recognize people who are always around, or with whom they've had a longstanding relationship, but will not be able to verbalize the people's names or any other information about them.

Language difficulties

Language ability is divided into expression and comprehension. With Alzheimer's disease, the ability to intelligibly express oneself with language tends to deteriorate faster than the ability to comprehend words and sentences. Most Alzheimer's patients have trouble finding the right words to express what they want to say. For example, a person might want to refer to his watch but can't remember the word "watch," so he says "the thing you tell time with." A person with Alzheimer's may also become confused and refer to her husband as her son or brother, mistaking one word for the other.

People in the mild stage of Alzheimer's disease are still able to have coherent conversations. They can also read out loud, understand what they're reading, and write sentences. In the moderate stage, they continue to be able to read and understand what they are reading, and comprehend what people say to them. But the ability to formulate coherent sentences and to name objects deteriorates. As it becomes more difficult to retrieve desired words, speech may become vague and imprecise. And as the ability to produce spontaneous sentences diminishes, the person may resort to repeating commonly used phrases over and over in a conversation.

In the severe stage, when many aspects of memory function are impaired and the person needs help with most activities of daily living, language comprehension and expression are both severely diminished. However, a person in the severe stage may still be able to recognize his or her name and respond when addressed directly. The ability to produce coherent sentences will vary from person to person. At this stage, some people with Alzheimer's disease do not speak at all.

Perception of time and orientation

Impaired orientation means that the person with Alzheimer's becomes increasingly confused about time (date, day of the week, month, year, season) and place (place of residence, neighborhood).

People in the mild stage may become confused about the date or day of the week. Time relationships may be slightly impaired. For example, people in the mild stage may get ready for an appointment hours ahead of time. Also, while it may be easy enough to navigate familiar places, such as their own neighborhood, unfamiliar locations begin to present a problem.

In the moderate stage, time orientation worsens. A person in this stage may believe that he or she is living in another period of life, and may think that deceased relatives are still alive. Orientation to place also declines. People in this stage will increasingly have trouble finding their way around, even in familiar places. They may not recall where to put items, such as the dishes or towels, and will store them in inappropriate locations. It's particularly important at this stage for people with Alzheimer's to be supervised and to have identification in case they become lost. (The Alzheimer's Association provides the "Safe Return" program, discussed in Chapter 8.)

Visual-spatial changes

Many people with Alzheimer's disease have problems with visual identification of objects and spatial orientation. A test often used to determine the extent of these problems is called the clock-drawing test. The person is asked to draw a clock with the hands set at a particular time. This task requires several cognitive abilities, including visual perception, spatial organizational ability, and planning. Some people with Alzheimer's disease are able to perform this task correctly, but many cannot.

Visual-spatial impairments also make it difficult to recognize faces and to identify and name objects. For example, a person with Alzheimer's disease may be unable to recall how common objects, such as a comb, toothbrush, or hammer, are used. The meaning of the object, not the skills involved in its use, are lost.

Visual-spatial changes also may account for some of the difficulties in driving—for example, not being able to accurately judge the size and shape of the car when parking, having small accidents that cause nicks and dents, and so forth.

The extent of disability with regard to visual-spatial ability depends on how much damage has been done to the area of the brain that controls this function.

Problem solving and judgment

One area that often becomes noticeably impaired is the ability to solve problems in day-to-day life. For example, a person with Alzheimer's disease may have trouble balancing her checkbook or handling a household emergency. She will also slowly lose the ability to grasp abstract concepts.

In the mild stage of Alzheimer's disease, impairments occur in problem-solving ability (such as doing calculations or managing complex tasks) and judgment. This is generally more of a problem with job-related functions at first. Even though the ability to deal with more than one task at a time becomes increasingly impossible, people in the mild stage can often continue to handle some household tasks, with the exception of financial transactions. The ability to handle finances, including checkbook management, bill payment, and understanding a bank statement, is already impaired in the mild stage of Alzheimer's disease. This capacity declines rapidly.

In the moderate stage, the person with Alzheimer's is not able to manage money at all. Before this happens, it is important that arrangements be made regarding the handling of finances (see Chapter 10, "Practical Advice"). This is especially important because cognitively impaired older adults can become victims of financial fraud schemes. Problem solving and judgment are generally impaired to the point where the person may not be able to handle a household emergency or make a decision about a stranger at the door.

Also in this stage, judgment about how to respond socially declines. It's not uncommon for people to act inappropriately in social situations, using coarse language or telling crude jokes. The enjoyment of social events and outings does not necessarily diminish. However, Alzheimer's patients may avoid social situations because of embarrassment about their condition and their inability to process new and complex information.

In the severe stage, problem solving and judgment are significantly impaired, and even simple decisions—such as what to eat and wear—must be supervised.

Mood and behavior changes

In addition to having impaired mental function, Alzheimer's patients may exhibit changes in mood and behavior. These can occur at any stage of the illness and tend to come and go. Mood and behavior changes vary widely from person to person.

Depression

Patients in the mild-to-moderate stage may become depressed. Generally, major depression is defined as a feeling of sadness and decreased interest in most things, most of the day, nearly every day, for at least two consecutive weeks. Other symptoms of major depression include:

- Decreased energy
- Change in appetite, often with weight loss
- Sleep disturbance
- Low self-esteem or guilt
- Decreased concentration
- Thoughts of suicide or the feeling that life is not worth living

Many depressed Alzheimer's patients do not experience all of the classic symptoms that occur in major depression. It may be difficult for a doctor to diagnose depression in people with Alzheimer's disease because some of the symptoms overlap. Nonetheless, depression in an Alzheimer's patient should be treated, often with antidepressant medication. Involvement in a support group may help early-stage patients counteract the symptoms of depression and social withdrawal.

Agitation and aggression

Some behavioral changes are also common. For example, a person with Alzheimer's disease may become more irritable than usual, getting angry without provocation. Agitation and aggression can develop, even in people who were easygoing prior to the illness, and people who were gregarious and outgoing may become subdued.

The behavioral changes, particularly agitation, can get more burdensome as the disease worsens. As language ability deteriorates, people with Alzheimer's may express agitation through behaviors such as screaming, pacing, and an inability to sit calmly. People in the moderate and later stages of Alzheimer's disease are likely to wander aimlessly from room to room.

Verbal or physical aggression may occur when a caregiver is helping with tasks such as bathing, grooming, or meal preparation. This may represent frustration over not being able to do these things independently or not comprehending the purpose of the tasks.

Sundowning

Sundowning—agitation that increases in the evening and night-time—is relatively common among people with Alzheimer's. It's not known why this happens, but people with this disturbance experience increased confusion, anxiety, agitation, and disorientation beginning at dusk and continuing throughout the night. Sundowning may be complicated by sleep disturbances. The person may sleep during the day and stay up all night.

This disruption in the normal cycle of sleeping at night and being awake in the daytime can be caused by an upset in the body's circadian rhythm (internal biological clock). It might also be due to other factors. Dim lights, increased shadows, and the lack of sensory cues from the immediate environment can cause confusion. Or, the person may be hungry, uncomfortable, or in pain and unable to appropriately express those needs.

Some strategies for dealing with sleep disturbances in people with Alzheimer's disease are described in Chapter 8, "Caring for a Person with Alzheimer's Disease."

Delusions and hallucinations

Some people with Alzheimer's disease experience delusions or hallucinations. A delusion is a false belief that is not consistent with reality. A hallucination is seeing, hearing, smelling, or feeling something that doesn't exist. Hallucinations are less common than delusions.

Some people with Alzheimer's disease who continually misplace objects—such as money, jewelry, keys, or even non-valuable items like papers, clothing, or cans of food—develop a paranoid delusion that someone has stolen them. They may become quite agitated about this concern. Sometimes people with Alzheimer's think that a deceased family member still lives in the house, or that strangers have moved in. Calm reassurance by a caregiver about the reality of the situation may alleviate these problems, at least temporarily.

The effect of Alzheimer's on day-to-day functioning

Household tasks

In the mild stage, people with Alzheimer's disease can generally continue to carry out their day-to-day tasks—going shopping, preparing meals, and doing household chores. Some supervision may be needed, and memory aids—such as lists, schedules, calendars, and alarms—may help to compensate for memory lapses. As memory problems worsen, more help will be needed. Simple tasks can continue to be performed, but anything requiring coordination of sequences of activities, such as home repair or car maintenance, will be problematic.

People in the moderate stage will require much more supervision. However, they can still do simple chores, such as washing dishes, setting the table, or making the bed. These involve the overly learned procedural memory system, which holds up the longest. Caregivers need to assess which tasks people are able to continue doing and which they need help with, and then allow them to continue to function at the highest possible level. The longer people can tend to household functions, the better it will be for their self-esteem and the longer they will be able to maintain some basic skills.

In the severe stage, the person with Alzheimer's will be unable to perform any household tasks, and will require complete assistance.

Involvement in the community

At first, Alzheimer's disease will not dramatically affect the person's ability to be involved in the community. He or she can still participate in senior groups and volunteer organizations, as well as usual recreational activities, such as playing cards or exercising.

In the moderate stage, it will become increasingly difficult to function independently. Participation in activities where appropriate direction is not available will become problematic. However, the person can still perform certain types of hobbies and recreational activities, and these should be encouraged. There are an increasing number of adult day care centers, including evening care programs and other supportive environments, where people with Alzheimer's disease can engage in meaningful activities under the necessary supervision. The social aspect of these programs is an important benefit.

In the severe stage, reliance on caregivers increases. However, many people with Alzheimer's disease continue to enjoy socializing in a supervised setting.

Personal care and grooming

In the beginning, people with Alzheimer's will be able to handle their own personal care (dressing, bathing, brushing teeth, shaving, eating). Although these activities involve judgment, planning, and visual-spatial skills, because they are highly practiced tasks, the memory of how to perform them remains intact for a while. However, difficulties with spatial relationships may make it necessary to have help tying shoelaces or buckling a belt.

In the moderate stage, there is wide variability in which functions remain and which require assistance. Some people continue to dress themselves, but it's likely that they will need help choosing what clothes to wear. Prompting may be necessary to ensure that clothes are put on in the correct order.

At this stage, help is often needed to bathe or take a shower. Shaving with an electric razor is usually preferable to using traditional razor blades. Brushing teeth and combing hair may or may not require assistance.

In the severe stages of Alzheimer's disease, help is needed with all personal care and grooming activities. Incontinence can occur, necessitating adult diapers and regular trips to the toilet. Some patients may require help cutting food, or they must be fed.

Driving

At some point, probably early on, it's best for a person with Alzheimer's disease to relinquish the car keys and stop driving. In the very early stage, some people will be able to continue driving without problems. However, the deficits that occur in Alzheimer's disease can impair critical functions and make driving dangerous. For example, a person with Alzheimer's disease may become disoriented (forgetting how to navigate to familiar places) or may react incorrectly in dangerous situations. Also, visual-spatial impairments and difficulty with problem solving and judgment may make the task of driving too challenging.

Giving up driving may be difficult to accept because it means losing a large degree of independence, particularly in suburban and rural areas that don't have public transportation systems. If you're unsure whether it's the right time for a person with Alzheimer's disease to stop driving, there are resources available to help with the decision.

The New York State Office for the Aging has published a handbook for families, friends, and caregivers who are worried about the safety of an aging driver (visit http://bit.ly/1uKbC8e). The handbook offers advice on how to assess an older driver's ability, and it is not specific to New York State. People living elsewhere can contact their state's office on aging to inquire about an older driver assessment program. You can also contact your physician or Department of Motor Vehicles to make arrangements for a road test.

Expected timeline of Alzheimer's

The duration of Alzheimer's disease from the mild stage to death varies widely from person to person, ranging from four to 20 years. Women with the disease tend to live somewhat longer than men. Compared to the overall U.S. population, people with Alzheimer's disease tend to have shorter life expectancies.

The progression of the disease is also highly individual. Caregivers need to pay close attention to activities and functions that the person with Alzheimer's disease is still capable of, and to encourage him or her to continue taking as active a role as possible in the day-to-day activities of living. There are caregiver training programs that provide instruction on how to help a loved one maintain personal skills.

TREATMENT

Despite reports of promising new therapies for Alzheimer's disease, there is still no cure. One or more of the drugs currently being tested may offer hope, but the results of those studies are still a few years away. In the meantime, there are drugs that can treat some of the symptoms. (see Box 7-1, "Alzheimer's drugs: essential facts"). These drugs may slow the rate of mental decline in many people with Alzheimer's disease. Mood and behavior symptoms—such as depression, agitation, anxiety, and delusions—can be managed with drugs and other therapies.

Alzheimer's disease drugs

Four main drugs are FDA-approved for Alzheimer's disease. Three of them—donepezil (Aricept), rivastigmine (Exelon), and galantamine (Razadyne)—are types of drugs called cholinesterase inhibitors. The fourth drug, memantine (Namenda), works by a different mechanism. A fifth drug, tacrine (Cognex), which is a cholinesterase inhibitor, is rarely used anymore due to its potential for detrimental effects on the liver.

Cholinesterase inhibitors

The plaques and tangles of Alzheimer's disease cause neurons in the brain to die, resulting in deteriorating brain function. Cholinesterase inhibitors don't stop neurons from dying. Instead, they help to boost the function of the cells that remain. Brain cells communicate via chemicals called neurotransmitters. Acetylcholine is a neurotransmitter that is depleted in the brains of people with Alzheimer's disease. Cholinesterase inhibitor drugs stop the enzyme cholinesterase from deactivating acetylcholine. In this way, more acetylcholine remains in the brain for mental functioning.

Studies have shown that the cholinesterase inhibitor drugs help about half of people who take them to maintain mental function without significant decline for approximately six months to two years. The drugs are generally considered to be most effective when given in the mild-to-moderate stages of Alzheimer's disease, but Aricept has also been FDA-approved for use in the later stages of the disease.

Cholinesterase inhibitor drugs can help to maintain brain function for a period of time, but once the function is lost it generally cannot

ALZHEIMER'S DRUGS: ESSENTIAL FACTS

MEDICATION	APPROVED FOR	DOSING
Donepezil (Aricept)	All stages	5 or 10 mg once a day
Rivastigmine (Exelon)	Mild to moderate	3 to 6 mg twice a day Skin patch, initial dose: 4.6 mg every 24 hours. Maintenance dose: 9.5 mg every 24 hours
Galantamine (Razadyne)	Mild to moderate	8 to 12 mg twice a day or 24 mg extended-release form once a day
Memantine (Namenda)	Moderate to severe	5 to 10 mg twice a day or 28 mg extended-release form once a day

be recovered. Because the drugs can't prevent neurons from dying, they don't stop the disease from worsening. And some people are not helped by these drugs at all.

People who do respond to cholinesterase inhibitors generally can retain their current level of memory, language ability, orientation, and attention for a longer period of time than if they were not taking the drugs. The drugs may also have beneficial effects on some behavioral symptoms, such as irritability, anxiety, apathy, and delusions. Studies also have shown that people with Alzheimer's who take the drugs are better able to handle daily self-care activities, thereby decreasing the amount of time caregivers must spend supervising them. People with Alzheimer's who take a cholinesterase inhibitor often can remain living at home longer before requiring nursing home care.

People who take these medications should have a positive response within three months. The only way to know if a cholinesterase inhibitor will help is to try it. The potential benefits, risks, costs, and side effects should be discussed beforehand with a doctor.

Aricept and the extended-release form of Razadyne are taken once a day, while Exelon and the short-acting form of Razadyne are taken twice a day. Exelon is also available in a skin patch, changed daily, which releases the drug slowly over time, eliminating the need for twice a day dosing. It also may cause fewer side effects than the pill form.

Side effects

Potential side effects of cholinesterase inhibitor drugs include nausea, diarrhea, vomiting, fatigue, and weight loss. These tend to be more of a problem at the highest doses of the medications or if the dosages are raised too quickly. If any of these side effects occur, consult your physician, who may reduce the dose or switch to a different drug.

Memantine for moderate to severe Alzheimer's

Memantine works on a different neurotransmitter than the cholinesterase inhibitors and appears to be helpful for people in the moderate-to-severe stages of Alzheimer's disease. This distinguishes it from the cholinesterase inhibitors, which are useful mainly in the mild-to-moderate stages. Rather than increasing levels of acetylcholine, memantine affects the neurotransmitter glutamate.

Glutamate plays an important role in the parts of the brain responsible for learning and memory. Too little of the neurotransmitter can impair learning and memory, but too much can have damaging effects on brain cells. Alzheimer's disease may be affected by both too much and too little glutamate at different times.

Memantine protects against excess glutamate and boosts levels of glutamate when they are too low. Possible side effects with memantine include headache, dizziness, confusion, and constipation, although the drug is usually well tolerated.

Because memantine works on a different neurotransmitter than the cholinesterase inhibitors, it can be taken together with one of these drugs. Adding memantine to the drug regimens of patients who were already taking donepezil further improved cognition, ability to perform daily activities, and overall function, according to an analysis of four large studies. Researchers have not tested all of the possible drug combinations. In addition, combination therapy for people in the mild stages of Alzheimer's has not been adequately tested.

Alternative treatments

Numerous herbal remedies, vitamins, and dietary supplements are touted as memory enhancers or treatments for Alzheimer's disease. Some of them may be modestly helpful. Many of them are readily available in drug and health food stores. But keep in mind that the claims about these products may not be based on scientific evidence. Dietary supplements and herbal remedies are not required to undergo the same rigorous study and review as prescription drugs. Therefore, they may not have undergone testing for the desired effect.

Some studies have been conducted to determine whether certain alternative treatments have an impact on Alzheimer's disease. For many of these the results have been negative or inconclusive. For example, coenzyme Q10 was considered a promising candidate based on studies in mice and in people with Parkinson's disease. Coenzyme Q10 has not been studied for its effectiveness in treating Alzheimer's disease. However, a study of a synthetic version of coenzyme Q10 (called idebenone) was conducted in Alzheimer's patients and found to have no effect.

The herb ginkgo biloba is often marketed as a memory enhancer. It acts as an antioxidant and also increases blood flow by dilating blood vessels. Some small studies suggested that people with Alzheimer's disease or another form of dementia had improved mental function when taking the herb. However, when ginkgo biloba was subjected to larger, more rigorous studies, it was no more effective than placebo (a sugar pill).

Overall, the evidence that ginkgo biloba improves mental function is weak, and any measurable effect is short lived. In addition, there may be some increased risk of bleeding with ginkgo use.

Antioxidants

Because damage from oxidation caused by free radicals has been observed in the brains of people with Alzheimer's disease, researchers have sought to discover whether taking antioxidant vitamins, such as vitamin E, has therapeutic value.

One study showed that patients in the moderate-to-severe stages of Alzheimer's disease who took 2,000 IU of vitamin E or 10 mg of selegiline (a drug used to control symptoms of Parkinson's disease) per day for two years were slower to lose their ability to perform basic daily living activities compared to similar patients who took a placebo.

Another study found that for people in earlier stages of Alzheimer's disease (mild to moderate) taking a daily dose of 2,000 IU of vitamin E slowed decline in the ability to engage in normal daily activities, which reduced some of the burden on caregivers.

These studies have caused some doctors to recommend that their Alzheimer's patients take 1,000 IU of vitamin E twice a day. It should be noted, however, that this is an extremely high dose. Taking such a high dose should be done only under the supervision of a doctor because there are potential adverse effects, such as an increased risk of bleeding.

As more research is conducted, it is important to consult your physician before taking large doses of any vitamins or other supplements.

Chinese herb: Huperzine A

A natural cholinesterase inhibitor, huperzine A, has similar properties as the cholinesterase inhibitor drugs donepezil, rivastigmine, and galantamine. Huperzine A, derived from the Chinese herb Huperzia serrata, is available without a prescription and is promoted as a memory enhancer. This herbal supplement has been used in Chinese traditional medicine for centuries, usually as a treatment for swelling, fever, and blood disorders. Chinese researchers have also found it may be useful for Alzheimer's disease.

Research suggests that this herb has an action similar to cholinesterase inhibitor drugs, which work by maintaining levels of the neurotransmitter acetylcholine in the brain. Acetylcholine is important for learning and memory.

A review of six small trials of huperzine A found that it appears to have some beneficial effects on improving mental function and reducing behavioral problems in people with Alzheimer's disease, with no obvious side effects. However, a larger trial of huperzine A in individuals with mild to moderate Alzheimer's disease found it was no better than placebo for improving mental function.

Because huperzine A is a natural herb, it doesn't need FDA approval in order to be sold, and thus the content of the pills you buy is not guaranteed. In addition, since it works on the same mechanism as the cholinesterase inhibitors, they should probably not be used together, as doing so would increase the risk of side effects.

Cognitive rehabilitation

It's often thought that damage to memory and learning systems in the brains of Alzheimer's patients makes it almost impossible to form new memories and learn new information. However, some researchers have rejected this idea and, using cognitive rehabilitation techniques, have tried to teach mildly to moderately impaired Alzheimer's disease patients to learn new information and improve their memories. These techniques can help teach people how to recall important information and to perform better in daily tasks.

Rehabilitation programs may involve learning face-name recognition techniques, getting memory notebooks in which to record appointments and schedules, and learning ways to improve financial skills. Two studies indicate that these techniques are effective. One group of researchers found that mildly impaired Alzheimer's disease patients who participated in three to four months of cognitive rehabilitation had a 170 percent improvement, on average, in their ability to recall faces and names, and a 71 percent improvement in their ability to provide proper change for a purchase. They were also able to process information more rapidly than similar patients who had not had the rehabilitation.

Another study showed that people in the early stage of Alzheimer's disease who participated in a cognitive rehabilitation program were able to retain implicit memories as well as younger adults and older adults without dementia. Implicit memory is the unconscious memory for common skills and activities, such as speaking a language or riding a bicycle.

Cognitive rehabilitation has traditionally been used to help people who've had strokes or suffered traumatic brain injuries recover cognitive functions and improve memory. Its use for Alzheimer's disease is relatively new, but the positive results from these studies show that people in the early stages of Alzheimer's disease can still learn, and this ability can be enhanced with cognitive rehabilitation techniques.

Treating behavioral symptoms

In addition to cognitive symptoms, people with Alzheimer's disease may exhibit behavioral symptoms, including anxiety, agitation, aggression, apathy, depression, delusions, and hallucinations. Drugs may help with some of these symptoms, but they are not always effective and can have undesirable side effects. Before medication is used, caregivers should try non-drug strategies. Recent evidence shows that physical exercise may help calm agitated behaviors in people with mild-to-moderate Alzheimer's disease (see Box 7-2, "Physical activity helpful for people with Alzheimer's disease").

Non-drug strategies

Changes in behavior often have specific causes, such as physical discomfort or pain that cannot be expressed, fear of unfamiliar surroundings and loud noises, frustration from trying to communicate with others, and annoyance at the inability to take care of household tasks and personal grooming. Moving to an assisted living facility or nursing home can cause agitation and other behavioral problems, as can changes in caregiver arrangements.

A person with Alzheimer's disease may be unable to describe specific physical complaints. Therefore, physical discomfort may be expressed as agitation. Look for evidence of common physical discomforts, such as pain, hunger, constipation, urinary tract infection, pneumonia, skin infection, or bone fracture. If present, these conditions should be appropriately treated.

New medical conditions or medications may also be sources of behavioral symptoms. For example, new or worsening vision or hearing problems can cause confusion or frustration. Many older adults, including those with Alzheimer's disease, take one or more prescription drugs for other health problems. Side effects from these drugs may affect behavior. When a new behavioral symptom occurs, look for a medical cause. A visit to the primary care doctor is recommended.

Once medical conditions have been addressed, there are other effective non-drug strategies that may help with some behavioral problems. For example, consistency in the home environment is important. The home should be arranged to reduce confusion, disorientation, and agitation. Lighting and noise levels should be adjusted to provide a calm environment (the lights shouldn't be so dim that they cause problems for people with low vision, however). Loud and erratic noises should be avoided. To make the home feel safe and to reduce anxiety, don't rearrange furniture or make any other drastic changes. Keep personal possessions, including favorite photographs, in visible locations, and don't move them around.

Handling agitation, irritability, and aggression

Caregivers can often lessen agitation, irritability, and aggression in a person with Alzheimer's disease by learning what to expect and how to communicate effectively. Sometimes breaking down a task into its component parts can decrease frustration and help the person to be more self-sufficient. For example, if a person with Alzheimer's disease gets agitated when asked to brush his teeth, break down the task into smaller directions. Say: "Take the toothbrush." "Put it under the water." "Here's the toothpaste." "Put the brush in your mouth." "OK, now you can brush."

Sometimes, the best remedy for agitation is gentle reassurance from a compassionate caregiver. People with Alzheimer's disease often mirror the emotions of those around them. If the caregiver becomes angry, agitated, or impatient, the person with dementia may pick up on these emotions and express them. If the caregiver is calm and reassuring, the person with dementia will pick up on that, and this may help.

Caregivers should help people with Alzheimer's disease plan activities, keep a schedule, and organize their time. Keeping the person involved in household and personal care activities for as long as possible may lessen feelings of helplessness and dependence. It's also important not to neglect leisure activities, such as music, painting, walking, or reading. Planning activities—both household and recreational—around a set schedule may help to relieve agitation.

Get support

Counseling and support groups are valuable resources for caregivers to discuss specific behaviors and get advice on how to handle them. The Alzheimer's Association has chapters across the United States that offer assistance and support groups, as well as a 24-hour helpline (see *Resources*, page 96).

Drug treatment

If non-drug strategies are not effective and symptoms of depression, anxiety, agitation, sleeplessness, and aggression are severe, a doctor may prescribe medications. Although there are no FDA-approved medications for the indication of behavioral disturbance from dementia, doctors have found that a variety of medications can be helpful to patients with these problems.

Antidepressants are designed to treat depression. The antidepressants most commonly used for older persons with dementia are from a group known as selective serotonin reuptake inhibitors (SSRIs), such as sertraline (Zoloft) or citalopram (Celexa). These drugs have relatively few side effects and are taken once a day. If they don't work, there are many other antidepressant drugs for the physician to choose from.

Anti-anxiety drugs may be used to relieve anxiety and help the person sleep. These include lorazepam (Ativan) and oxazepam (Serax). Drugs may be given over the short term to calm a person down during a crisis, or they may be given as needed for longer periods to deal with more persistent problems. All of the drugs used for behavioral symptoms have benefits and potential side effects, including risk for falling, and patients who are taking them need to be carefully monitored.

Antipsychotic drugs are sometimes used to treat agitation, hallucinations, and delusions in people with Alzheimer's disease. These drugs may be helpful for some people in certain circumstances, but they must be used with extreme caution. Some of the antipsychotic drugs can cause side effects, such as sedation, confusion, and weight gain. In addition, all antipsychotics may increase the risk for death among people with dementia. The FDA has issued a warning about this possibility.

Antipsychotics may be appropriate for some people in some circumstances. For example, they may be effective for people with severe agitation. Antipsychotic drugs should most likely be used only as a last resort and for the shortest possible time at the lowest possible dose. They should not be used to sedate or restrain a person.

It may take several attempts to find the right drug, or combination of drugs, that are most helpful. Even if drugs are used for behavioral symptoms, it is important to continue using non-drug approaches to calm agitated and irritable behavior.

CARING FOR A PERSON WITH ALZHEIMER'S DISEASE

If a loved one has Alzheimer's disease and you will be the primary caregiver, there's much you need to know, both about how to care for the person with the condition and about how to care for yourself. More than half of the people with Alzheimer's disease are cared for at home. This chapter will review some general information about caring for a person with Alzheimer's disease. The next next chapter is about services for the caregiver.

First and foremost, you should know that there are many resources available to help you, and you should avail yourself of as many of them as you need. Several helpful agencies are listed in *Resources*, on page 96. One in particular is the Alzheimer's Association—a nonprofit organization dedicated to providing education and support for people diagnosed with the condition, as well as for their families and care-givers. The Alzheimer's Association has a network of support groups throughout the United States. They can be extremely helpful in a number of ways. For one thing, you will feel less alone. You are not the only person coping with a difficult transition in your life. Over 15 million Americans are currently providing unpaid care for a person with Alzheimer's disease or another form of dementia, according to the Alzheimer's Association.

Once a person is diagnosed with Alzheimer's disease, he or she will require increasing amounts of assistance with daily life. This help can come from a spouse, child, other close family member, friend, or paid caregiver. One person can manage this task in the mild stage of the condition. As the disease progresses, however, additional help, and more outside services, will be needed. This chapter will review some care options, such as adult day services, respite care, in-home care, and nursing home care, and will offer suggestions to help you care for a person with Alzheimer's disease.

Care options

Most people with Alzheimer's disease live at home, with care provided by family and friends. But there are other care options. The living situation for each individual will depend to a large extent on the current family situation.

According to the Alzheimer's Association, about 800,000 people with Alzheimer's disease (more than one in seven) live alone. A person with Alzheimer's disease who lives alone with no family close by may be able to manage for a while in the mild stage of the disease. But the person will need to be taken in by a family member, have in-home care, or move to an assisted living facility or nursing home before the disease makes living alone dangerous. People with Alzheimer's disease can put themselves in danger in several ways, such as forgetting to turn off the stove, opening the door to a stranger who may rob them, forgetting to eat, or scalding themselves with hot water.

If the person with Alzheimer's disease is living with a spouse, child, or another adult who has good mental function and is in reasonably good health, it's possible to remain in the home. At some point, a home health aide may be needed (part-time or full-time) to help with care. If the person with Alzheimer's disease is being cared for at home, respite care services may be helpful for providing relief for the caregiver and to give the patient a social outlet.

Adult day services

Adult day services, which serve adults who are physically or cognitively impaired, are one type of respite care. This is a place where people with Alzheimer's disease can come for part of the day to interact socially and engage in recreational activities in a safe and supportive environment.

Adult day services offer caregivers a chance to go to their job or have free time without worrying about the safety of their loved one. Adult day programs offer people with Alzheimer's disease a place where they can interact with other people, receive services such as physical or speech therapy, and get some exercise.

Most adult day services will pick up and drop off participants and provide nursing care, personal care, counseling, therapeutic activities, and rehabilitation therapies. These may include reminiscence groups, exercise classes, arts and crafts, and music therapy. A meal is usually provided, as well as assistance with daily activities.

The number of adult day services has been growing over recent years to meet the increasing demand. To find one in your area, look in the Yellow Pages (under adult day care, adult day services, or senior citizen services), contact the Area Agency on Aging (call 800-677-1116), contact a local senior center, or ask your doctor.

Adult day programs are offered by hospitals, nursing homes, senior centers, and religious, fraternal, and neighborhood organizations. Depending on the type of organization providing the service, the cost can vary widely. Some programs may use a sliding scale or even be free. Adult day services are not covered by Medicare, but they may be covered by Medicaid or private long-term care insurance.

Once you've identified one or more adult day services, you should do some investigation (some questions to ask are listed in Box 8-1, "Questions to ask an adult day service provider"). It's also a good idea to pay a visit and see for yourself whether it meets the needs of your loved one. Look for a clean and pleasant atmosphere with sturdy, comfortable furniture. Watch the staff interact with participants. You may want to try out the service for three or four days before making a longer-term commitment.

Because an adult day service is an unfamiliar setting, it will probably take several visits before a person with Alzheimer's disease feels comfortable there. The caregiver may want to accompany him the first few times until he adjusts.

Longer-term respite care

There can be times when you are unable to carry out caregiving tasks for several days. For example, an emergency may arise or you may go on vacation. For these times, many nursing homes or assisted-living facilities offer respite care programs, usually for up to three weeks. You can find a respite care program in your area by contacting your local chapter of the Alzheimer's Association or the Area Agency on Aging.

In-home care

Home care services can fulfill duties ranging from helping with housework to providing skilled nursing care. In the mild stage of the disease, a homemaker or chore worker may be hired to do housekeeping, meal preparation, and shopping. The caregiver also can accompany the person to appointments, the movies, or other activities. These workers don't provide hands-on care, but they do make it possible for people with Alzheimer's disease to continue functioning independently for a longer period of time.

Home health aides are the next level up of care. They assist patients with daily activities, such as bathing, dressing, eating, and using the toilet. Home health aides are not nurses, but they are usually required to receive training and to work under the supervision of a nurse. Depending on the individual needs of a person with Alzheimer's, home health aides may be necessary from a few hours a day to 24 hours a day, seven days a week.

In-home caregivers can be hired privately or through a home health agency. You can get a referral from your physician or social worker, check the Yellow Pages, or contact the Area Agency on Aging.

BOX 8-1

Questions to ask an adult day service provider

☑ Is it open the days and hours you need it?

☑ Is transportation provided?

☑ Is it state-licensed or certified?

☑ Are there any conditions that would preclude your loved one from being accepted (for example, incontinence or being in a wheelchair)?

☑ How many staff members are there for how many participants? A good staff-to-participant ratio is one to four.

☑ What types of activities are offered? Make sure these are activities you think the Alzheimer's patient would enjoy.

☑ Are the meals nutritious and tasty?

☑ How much does it cost?

Also, the National Association for Home Care & Hospice has a Home Care Locator on their website (www.nahc.org), which lists home care agencies across the U.S. In 2012, the average hourly rate for home health aides was $21 ($168 for an eight-hour day), according to the MetLife Market Survey of Nursing Home, Assisted Living, Adult Day Services and Home Care Costs. For homemaker or companion services, the average hourly rate was $20.

Some states require home care agencies to be licensed and to meet minimum standards. If your state has these requirements, check to see if the home care agency you're considering is licensed.

In most cases, the cost of home care is borne by the patient and family. Medicare, Medicaid, and most health insurance plans have strict guidelines for covering home health care, and many Alzheimer's patients do not qualify. Long-term care insurance will cover home care if the patient and caregivers meet certain criteria.

Housing options

At some point between the mild and severe stage of the disease, it may make sense for the person with Alzheimer's to move to an assisted-living facility or nursing home. The decision to move someone to one of these facilities is rarely easy. The timing will depend on individual circumstances. A person living alone will need to move to the safety of an assisted-living facility or nursing home sooner than someone who has a caregiver at home. For the caregiver, the decision is more complex.

Caregiving can be very stressful. Some people move a loved one when caregiving becomes overly burdensome. This may be when the person with Alzheimer's becomes incontinent or behaviors become unmanageable.

One study found that counseling can help caregivers better cope with memory and behavior problems, which relieves some of the stress of caregiving. Receiving this type of counseling often delays the need to place the person in a nursing home. This is significant, in part because of the high cost of nursing home care. Rates for assisted-living facilities are less, but the cost is still high.

Nevertheless, it might eventually become necessary to move the person with Alzheimer's disease to an assisted-living facility or nursing home. Which facility is most appropriate will depend on the person's health. A person with few medical problems aside from Alzheimer's disease can live in an assisted-living facility that is set up to accommodate residents with dementia. If the person has other medical problems, placement in a nursing home may be the better option.

Selecting an assisted-living facility or nursing home can be difficult. Just as with choosing an adult day service, you need to thoroughly check out the facilities you are considering. Get recommendations from your physician, social worker, clergy, family, or friends. Visit each facility and ask questions (see Box 8-2, "Questions to ask when evaluating assisted-living facilities and nursing homes"). The Medicare website has detailed information about the past performance of every Medicare and Medicaid certified nursing home in the country (http://1.usa.gov/YAtMPK).

Assisted-living facilities

Assisted-living facilities were first conceived to provide healthy older adults with an essentially independent, but communal living environment. They rent a room or apartment and provide meals, along with housekeeping and laundry services, but they do not offer nursing services. Depending on the facility, assistance with daily activities, such as bathing and dressing, may be available. An assisted-living facility may be acceptable for a healthy person in the mild stage of Alzheimer's disease.

Some assisted-living facilities also have sections specifically designed for people with Alzheimer's disease. They offer a safe environment, special assistance for people with the disease, and appropriate activities. An assisted-living facility with a designated Alzheimer's unit can usually accept people at any stage of the disease if they are otherwise reasonably healthy.

A word of caution: Assisted-living facilities are not as closely monitored as nursing homes. They are not necessarily state-licensed, and regulations vary from state to state. The quality of the facilities and of the care varies widely. Take the time to thoroughly investigate a facility before choosing it, and make sure it's licensed. Also, make sure the facility is in compliance with all state regulations. Contact your state office on the aging to find out what laws and regulations apply.

In addition to taking an official tour of the facility, show up unannounced and observe the conditions on your own. When choosing an assisted-living facility, you'll be given a contract to sign. Show the contract to a lawyer who has expertise in elder law before signing.

The average monthly cost for a private, one-bedroom unit in an assisted living residence was $3,550 ($42,600 a year) in 2012 (the most recent year for which data are available), according to the "MetLife Market Survey of Nursing Home, Assisted Living, Adult Day Services, and Home Care Costs." The pricing can be complex and dependent on the services the resident needs. Assisted-living residences that provide

BOX 8-2

Questions to ask when evaluating assisted-living facilities and nursing homes

- ☑ Is it clean?
- ☑ How is medical care provided?
- ☑ How does the staff seem to relate to the residents?
- ☑ Is there a good staff-to-resident ratio?
- ☑ Is there a special Alzheimer's unit?
- ☑ Are patients' personal belongings in the rooms?
- ☑ What are the visiting hours?
- ☑ What is the policy on taking the resident out of the facility for short visits with family and friends?

specialized dementia care often charge additional monthly fees. Long-term health insurance does not cover assisted living, and you can't count on Medicaid to pay the bill. Although in certain states, Medicaid will pay for some services provided in an assisted-living facility, the overall cost is borne by the individual.

Nursing homes

Skilled nursing facilities (nursing homes) offer the highest level of care and may be appropriate for people in the moderate or severe stages of Alzheimer's disease. They provide 24-hour nursing care and supervision, including help with bathing and grooming, medical and nursing care, and activities.

Many nursing homes have added separate special-care units to meet the needs of people with dementia. The living spaces in these units will have features such as secured exits, single-occupancy rooms, small dining rooms, and designated indoor and outdoor areas for wandering. Activities accommodate the cognitive deficits of people with Alzheimer's.

In 2012, the average cost for a private room in a nursing home was $90,520 per year and the average cost for a semi-private room was $81,030, according to the "MetLife Market Survey of Nursing Home, Assisted Living, Adult Day Services, and Home Care Costs." For those who are eligible, Medicaid will help pay the cost, but it can be difficult to qualify for Medicaid if you have financial assets. Speak to an elder-care lawyer to learn about your rights and benefits.

Once you've made a choice and moved your loved one into an assisted-living facility or nursing home, you need to maintain an active presence. Even though nursing homes are required to meet certain standards, it's a good idea to continue to oversee the patient's care.

Geriatric care managers

Understanding the various care options and making decisions about what is best for a loved one can overwhelm family members of a person with Alzheimer's disease. Professional assistance is available. Geriatric care managers are professionals (usually social workers) who can be hired to assist in a number of ways. Care managers—who usually charge $50 to $200 per hour—can perform an assessment of a person in their home and devise strategies to keep them safe and help compensate for some of the memory problems. They can also assist with hiring caregivers and can act as liaison to family members living far away.

A geriatric care manager can also help to determine if assisted living or nursing care is necessary. They can provide a one-time assessment and recommendations, or they can oversee care over the long term. To find a geriatric care manager in your area, contact the National Association of Professional Geriatric Care Managers (www. caremanager.org).

If you can't afford a geriatric care manager, contact your local office on aging for help. They may be able to send a case manager to do an assessment at no charge. To find the agency near you, enter your zip code at the website www.eldercare.gov.

The challenges of caregiving

As a person with Alzheimer's disease loses the ability to function in certain ways, he or she will increasingly require help. In general, the caregiver must be the patient's advocate, ensuring his or her safety, medical well-being, and financial security. The caregiver must assist with day-to-day activities and provide emotional support. Caregivers must compensate for the patient's cognitive problems and cope with the behavioral problems.

In the mild stage, people with Alzheimer's disease can usually manage on their own, provided that someone checks on them regularly (at least once a day). However, they will most likely need help with finances, and they may need someone to do the grocery shopping. As the disease progresses, they will need increasing assistance with household activities.

In the moderate stage, living alone is no longer an option. Assistance will be required with grooming, dressing, meal preparation, and household chores. The most care is required in the severe stage.

Caregiving can be challenging in a number of ways. For people with Alzheimer's disease, the growing loss of independence and privacy can be very frustrating, and even depressing. They may express their frustration by resisting help and insisting that they are still capable of doing things, even if they aren't.

Some people with Alzheimer's disease become suspicious of the very people who are trying to help them, especially those who are taking over financial responsibilities. This is understandable, given the mental changes that occur in people with Alzheimer's.

When dealing with troublesome or confusing behaviors, it's helpful to think about the situation from the perspective of the person with the cognitive impairment. This will help you find appropriate ways to respond that don't exacerbate the problem. It will also help you come up with creative memory aids and other methods to help the person compensate for cognitive deficits.

Some resources, including books, manuals, and instructional videos, to help caregivers work with people with dementia are available from the Center for Applied Research in Dementia (see Resources, page 96). They developed memory techniques for people with Alzheimer's disease based on an education system called Montessori, which was first developed for young children. Using these techniques, caregivers assist people with Alzheimer's disease to make the most of the skills and habits they have retained, such as singing, playing a musical instrument, playing golf, or any other activity that engages the person. The key is to personalize the program by identifying activities, hobbies, and skills that the person enjoys and finding ways to continue these activities, possibly in a modified fashion. Memory exercises, such as sorting items into categories and matching colored balls to cups, may help to improve memory for some people.

Communication

As Alzheimer's disease worsens, communication will become more difficult, but not impossible. It's very important to talk with your spouse, parent, or friend and find out directly from them how you can assist them. This will be easier in the mild stage of the disease, but it's important to continue communicating throughout the course of the illness. Even in the severe stage, a person with Alzheimer's disease will still want to communicate.

Keep in mind that people with Alzheimer's disease can generally comprehend more than they can express with language. If your loved one is having difficulty finding the right words to express a thought, it doesn't mean she can't understand you if you offer suggestions. Also, remember that spoken language is only one form of communication. Body language, tone of voice, and facial expressions are all aspects of communication that help get a message across.

Language difficulties will vary among people with Alzheimer's disease. Some common problems include: being unable to find the right words, using the same words repeatedly, having difficulty forming sentences correctly, inventing words for familiar objects, and speaking less often.

Given these problems, it often takes patience to understand what a person with Alzheimer's disease is trying to convey. Listen carefully and try to get as many nonverbal cues as possible. Give the person time to think and describe what he wants. If he's having trouble finding the right words, offer suggestions. But avoid telling him he's wrong. Instead, repeat what you think he's trying to say for clarification. If you still don't understand, you can ask him to point or gesture. It's also helpful to try to get a sense of the emotions behind the words. Sometimes the person's feelings are more essential to what's being communicated than the actual words.

When speaking to someone with Alzheimer's disease, there are some ways to accommodate cognitive deficits. Speak in a calm voice, look the person in the eye, and use short and concise sentences. The person may forget what you've just said, so repeat yourself patiently when necessary. When giving the person directions, break up the task into one-step instructions. Tell them one step at a time. Frame questions so that they require only a yes or no answer or have multiple choices. For example, don't say, "What would you like for dinner?" Instead, say, "Would you like chicken or fish for dinner?"

Avoid dictating to the person or overloading her with information. And don't argue or criticize. This can cause confusion, fear, and anxiety.

If the person with Alzheimer's disease has an angry outburst, don't take it personally. This is often caused by feelings of frustration. Try to determine the cause of the frustration, and reassure the person as much as possible. Tell her not to worry about something she's forgotten to do or her inability to find a misplaced item. Using kind words, tell her she's not alone and that you are there to help her.

In the later stages of the disease, communication remains important, even though verbal skills are considerably impaired. Sharing time with nonverbal activities, such as listening to music, dancing, looking at photographs, or holding hands, may substitute for conversation.

Sometimes communication is hindered by poor vision or impaired hearing. Make sure the Alzheimer's patient has her vision and hearing regularly tested, and that she gets glasses or a hearing aid if necessary.

Memory and reminiscence aids

Memory aids are generally helpful in the mild stage of Alzheimer's disease. There are no standard aids that work for everyone. A person with Alzheimer's disease will probably have to try out different memory tricks to see what helps.

Some people carry around a notebook with the names and phone numbers of people they often call. The notebook may also contain written reminders about chores, and instructions for doing tasks. Some people leave written reminders in strategic places around the house—for example, a note on the washing machine with step-by-step instructions for turning it on. Other people find that labeling things is helpful. Written signs may be placed around the house that read "refrigerator," "sock drawer," "bathroom," etc. Also, place a calendar on the wall and mark off the days to make it easier to remember the day and date.

These memory aids will facilitate day-to-day tasks. It's also important to have cues for remembering key people and events in the person's life. Keep favorite photographs, newspaper clippings, and other things that are meaningful to the patient in prominent locations around the home, or on a bulletin board. You might also want to make a book with pictures and other mementos of important people and events from the past.

Bathing, dressing, and other daily activities

In the moderate and severe stages of the disease, a person with Alzheimer's will need more help with basic hygiene and grooming, such as bathing, dressing, and dental care. This may be difficult. People with dementia resist assistance with personal care for a number of reasons. They might not want anyone intruding on their privacy. Also, the process of bathing and dressing can become too complicated and confusing. A person with Alzheimer's might not remember when she last took a bath and insist that she doesn't need one.

To smooth the way for a problem-free bath, try to prepare everything in advance. Run the bath water, have towels nearby, make the room temperature comfortable. Then give the person one-step instructions: "It's time for a bath." "Unbutton your shirt." "Now take off your pants." "Step into the bathtub." If the person is self-conscious about being naked, respect her dignity. Allow her to hold a towel in front of her body when getting in and out of the tub or shower. Make sure there are non-slip adhesives on the floor of the tub and a grab bar to prevent falls.

Try to maintain the bathing routine the patient has already established. If she's always bathed in the morning right before breakfast, keep to that schedule. If bathing becomes difficult, don't require her to take a bath every day. Sometimes a sponge bath can substitute if you meet with insurmountable resistance.

When it comes to dressing, keep clothing choices simple. Help the person pick out coordinated clothes and then lay them out in the order they are to be put on. If necessary, give the person short instructions. When purchasing new clothes, think about comfort and simplicity. Shirts that button in the front are sometimes easier than pullover tops. If buttons and zippers are too difficult to manage, try replacing them with Velcro. Slip-on shoes are easier than shoes with laces.

People with Alzheimer's also will eventually need help with oral hygiene. As the disease progresses, brushing and flossing teeth will become difficult. Rather than telling the person to brush her teeth, you may need to break it down into smaller steps: "Hold your toothbrush." "Put toothpaste on your toothbrush." You may need to demonstrate for her. Regular trips to the dentist continue to be important for a person with Alzheimer's disease. Inform the dentist of the person's condition ahead of time. You may need to search around to find a dentist who has experience working with people who have Alzheimer's.

Wandering

Wandering is very common among people with Alzheimer's disease, and it can be dangerous if the person wanders out of the house and gets lost. There are a number of strategies to deal with wandering. First, safeguard the house to make it less likely that the person will wander out the front door. For example:

▶ Place an alarm on the doorknob.
▶ Use childproof doorknob covers.
▶ Paint doors the same color as surrounding walls, making it more difficult for the person with dementia to identify the door.
▶ Install motion-activated alarms, which trigger an alarm if the person crosses a line, thus breaking an infrared beam.

Enroll the person in the Alzheimer's Association's "Safe Return" program. This program provides an identification bracelet, necklace, clothing tags, and wallet cards with contact information in case the person is found wandering. Make sure you have a recent photo available in case it is needed to help find someone who has wandered.

A high-tech solution to keeping track of a loved one with dementia is also available from the Alzheimer's Association. Called ComfortZone, this internet-based system provides information on a person's location. The person wears or carries a GPS device, which receives signals from satellites or cell towers. Family members can access information about the person's location from a web site. They can request alerts when the person leaves a specified zone or use the device only in an emergency. The device costs $100 to $200 and there is an additional monthly fee depending on the type of plan chosen.

Sometimes people wander because they're bored, restless, or confused. One way to reduce wandering is to keep the person with Alzheimer's engaged in activities. Go for walks or include the person in simple household chores, such as folding laundry.

Sleep problems

People with Alzheimer's disease are at increased risk of having disturbed sleep. They can become agitated and disoriented and stay awake all night. Medical experts don't fully understand why sleep disturbances occur in Alzheimer's disease, but there are some theories. It might simply be that the person hasn't had enough activity during the day to be tired at night, or that older adults in general need less sleep than do younger people. Also, nighttime is associated with increased confusion, which leads to agitation that interferes with going to sleep. In addition, there may be a disturbance in the internal biological clock, which upsets the normal sleep/wake cycle.

To combat nighttime sleeplessness, keep the person with Alzheimer's busy during the day. Refrain from offering caffeinated beverages in the evening. There are also medications that can help with nighttime agitation and sleep disturbances.

Researchers have looked into ways to readjust the sleep/wake cycle. Exposing the person to bright light early in the morning (thus cueing the body that it is morning and time to be awake), restricting the amount of time spent in bed, and using the over-the-counter remedy melatonin (a substance naturally produced by the body to regulate sleep/wake cycles) have been shown in studies to be helpful.

For safety, put nightlights in the bedroom and bathroom to avoid falls in the middle of the night. Restrict access to rooms by locking doors or installing safety gates. Install door sensors to alert people in the house that the person is awake.

If you want to coax the person back to sleep, speak calmly and remind him of the time. Ask if he's up because he needs to use the bathroom or if he wants something. If he won't go back to bed, but will fall asleep on a couch or in a lounge chair, allow him to do that.

Exercise

Exercise, such as brisk walking, has demonstrated benefits for both physical and mental health in people with dementia. It can reduce physical decline, frailty, and falls.

An analysis of 30 studies on the effects of exercise on people with cognitive impairment confirms this. Exercise was found to increase overall fitness and mental function, and to have a positive impact on behavior in people with dementia. One study showed that people with Alzheimer's disease had a slower rate of decline in physical functioning if they engaged in an exercise regimen. This physical activity resulted in fewer falls, which translated to savings in healthcare costs. Therefore, regular walks of 20 to 60 minutes with a companion should be part of a routine for as long as the patient is able.

Maximize existing function

In part, a caregiver's job is to help people with Alzheimer's disease carry out tasks they can no longer manage. But it's equally important to encourage them to continue doing things they are still able to do, and to find creative ways to help them compensate for cognitive deficits. For example, a person who's lost the ability to communicate effectively with speech may be better able to communicate in other ways, such as through music or art. Music and art therapists can help bring out a patient's musical or artistic side.

Conclusion

Caring for a person with Alzheimer's disease can be a challenging and complex task, and caregivers need constant information and support. The Alzheimer's Association offers support groups, workshops, and written materials for caregivers. The more acquainted you become with strategies for handling the changes that occur, the easier it will be for you to offer loving and supportive care.

HANDLING CAREGIVER STRESS

BOX 9-1

Typical responses to caregiving

- Guilt
- Anger
- Financial strain
- Fatigue
- Neglect of one's own health
- Depression
- Sleep disturbances
- Social isolation
- Difficulty dealing with the loss of shared memories

When a family member or close friend has Alzheimer's disease, the focus of attention naturally shifts to the needs of the person with the condition. Decisions must be made about living arrangements, caregiving, and financial and legal matters. The people who will be caregivers must learn how best to assist the person as the disease continues to worsen.

While it's certainly important to do everything you can to be a helpful advocate and caregiver, it's equally important not to neglect yourself. Caregiving can be time-consuming and stressful. The stress may be compounded by financial strain, because many services required by people with Alzheimer's disease are not covered by Medicare or health insurance.

As your caregiving role increases, you may have less free time, experience frequent interruptions at work, and find it hard to deal with your own health and interests. You might have trouble sleeping. At times you may feel angry, lonely, bitter, and resentful (see Box 9-1, "Typical responses to caregiving"). These are normal feelings, and you shouldn't feel guilty about having them. It's helpful to have a support group, such as close friends and family; a church, synagogue or other spiritual community; or an organized support group of caregivers. By expressing your emotions among supportive individuals, you're less likely to take them out on the patient. Support groups also can be valuable sources of information, and they offer a safe and accepting environment in which to share your experiences.

Counseling for caregivers

You might also consider seeking individual counseling with a social worker or psychologist. For many people, the stress of caregiving can be exhausting. For some it leads to depression when the demands of caregiving become overwhelming. This is not unusual; nearly half of all caregivers become depressed at some time.

Many people reach a point at which they simply can't handle the stress and must move their loved one to a nursing home or other facility. Researchers have found, however, that caregivers who receive support and counseling not only are able to keep the Alzheimer's patient home longer, but they are also less stressed.

One study found that Alzheimer's patients whose spouses received counseling and support were able to remain at home for 1.5 years longer before being placed in a nursing home than patients whose spouses did not receive counseling. The caregivers who had access to counseling and support were better able to tolerate the patients' memory and behavior problems, were more satisfied with support from family and friends, and had fewer symptoms of depression. A follow-up to this study found that spouse caregivers who received counseling and support were better able to preserve their own health.

Caregivers often have a tendency to neglect their own health. In addition to depression, caregiver stress can make people susceptible to other medical problems, such as hypertension, irritable bowel syndrome, migraines, heart problems, and ulcers. One study found that older adults caring for a family member with dementia were at higher risk for cognitive impairment and dementia themselves. That's why it's important for you to keep up with regular doctor visits. Continue to eat a healthy diet, get plenty of rest, and exercise regularly. Consider simple exercises, such as brisk walking, swimming, or jogging, on most days of the week (see Box 9-2, "How caregivers can help themselves").

Caregiver stress

How you deal with the stress of caregiving will depend to some degree on your personality and the way you cope with stress. People with a take-charge attitude may experience less stress, for example. However, the complexities of caregiving can make coping difficult for just about anyone.

A need to learn new skills might magnify your stress. For example, a husband may have to learn to cook and manage his wife's former household tasks. If the spouse who handled the finances and wrote the checks is the one to develop Alzheimer's disease, the other partner might have to take a quick course in basic finances.

Above all, don't try to do everything yourself. Caregiving is too big a job for one person. Get the help you need from family, friends, home attendants, support groups, adult day programs, and respite care. Find out what resources are available in your community from senior centers or your local agency on aging. Ask family and friends to visit and help out. Getting support will help both you and your loved one feel less socially isolated. Working together will help ensure that the person with Alzheimer's gets the best possible care.

Caregiving doesn't have to be a negative experience. In fact, many people derive an increased sense of purpose from their new

BOX 9-2

How caregivers can help themselves

- Develop a daily schedule.
- Set aside time for yourself.
- Coordinate caregiving tasks among different family members and friends.
- Engage in relaxing activities on a daily basis.
- Attend a support group or individual counseling sessions.
- Maintain a social network.
- Hire professional caregivers to help when necessary.
- Consider day programs or long-term-care placement, if appropriate.

responsibilities, and they grow emotionally. Take care of yourself, take one day at a time, and allow people to help you. Focus on and enjoy what your loved one can still do. Perhaps most importantly, don't lose your sense of humor. A little humor can get you through some rough situations, and it makes life a lot more fun. Alzheimer's disease doesn't remove a person's sense of humor. So laugh with your loved one. You'll both enjoy it.

PRACTICAL ADVICE: LEGAL, FINANCIAL, HEALTH CARE

BOX 10-1

Receiving a diagnosis of Alzheimer's disease for yourself or a loved one may be upsetting, and practical matters may not be the first thing on your mind. But at some point early in the disease, it's very important to make certain legal and financial decisions and to think about future care. Even if a person with Alzheimer's disease is still capable of handling his own affairs, this will eventually change. Making legal and financial decisions early allows the person to actively participate in the planning of his or her own future. The decisions need to be set down in legal documents at a time when the person is still mentally competent enough to make decisions (see Box 10-1, "Checklist of legal documents you should draw up—before it's too late"). Having a diagnosis of Alzheimer's disease does not, by itself, mean that a person is incapable of making fundamental decisions. But there will come a time when the person's decision-making ability will end.

Legal planning

Start by consulting a lawyer who is familiar with trusts, estates, and laws pertaining to Medicare/Medicaid. Ask for a referral to someone who is experienced in elder or geriatric law. Your local Commission on Aging or your local Alzheimer's Association chapter may be able to help as well. You need to have a will, and you will have to establish procedures for how financial and health care decisions will be made. Laws vary from state to state. If you're helping a relative who lives in another state, retain a lawyer who has expertise in the laws of the state in which the person with Alzheimer's lives.

Many people choose to grant "power of attorney" to a trusted family member or friend, who will take care of legal and financial transactions. However, a simple power of attorney is not enough because it becomes void when the person granting it is mentally incapable of making decisions. Therefore the situation requires "durable power of attorney." This authorizes the designated person to act on behalf of someone who is unable to make his or her own decisions.

You might also want to consider setting up a living trust. Assets are put into a trust, and a trustee (an individual or bank) will be responsible for managing the trust when the individual is no longer able.

When it comes to making arrangements for future medical decisions, you have basically two options: a health care proxy (also called

---

Checklist of legal documents you should draw up— before it's too late

☑ Durable power of attorney

☑ Living trust

☑ Living will

☑ Healthcare proxy

ADVICE: BE PREPARED...

☑ Get informed on Medicaid and Medicare policies at the onset of Alzheimer's disease.

☑ Purchase long-term care insurance before the actual diagnosis—or it may be too late.

☑ Get informed about tax issues regarding Alzheimer's disease. You may be eligible for some tax breaks.

a power of attorney for health care) and a living will. A health care proxy is a person you designate to make decisions on your behalf if you can no longer speak for yourself—often the same person to whom you would give durable power of attorney. This includes making decisions about medical treatment and eventually end-of-life decisions, such as whether to use a respirator to prolong life. When choosing a health care proxy, make sure it is someone you trust, and that he or she is willing to accept the responsibility. Also, have a conversation with your proxy and family members about your wishes.

A living will lets you state your wishes about medical care in advance, in the event that you later become unable to communicate. This is more limited than naming a health care proxy, because it is very difficult to anticipate specific health problems in advance. But a living will may be used to make your wishes clear about the use of artificial life support systems. The laws about living wills vary from state to state, so check with your lawyer to determine how best to express your wishes for future medical care.

If the proper legal documents are not set up before the person becomes mentally incompetent to sign them, it is necessary to go to court to have a judge appoint someone to act as guardian. The guardian then has the legal authority to make certain decisions on the patient's behalf. This process is time-consuming and costly, and it involves a court proceeding before a judge. It can be avoided with some advance planning.

Financial planning

Once Alzheimer's disease worsens, the ability to handle finances deteriorates. Additionally, providing care for a person with Alzheimer's disease is often costly. When considering the management of your financial affairs and the payment for your care, you should discuss the options with an attorney, a financial planner or an accountant—someone well versed in Medicare and Medicaid rules and regulations.

Begin with an assessment of your personal assets, including your financial resources and sources of income. Resources include bank and credit union accounts, investments (stocks and bonds), life insurance, health insurance, and real estate. Sources of income may be from salary, retirement benefits, Social Security, veterans' benefits, rental income, interest, and dividends. Next, list any financial liabilities, such as loans, credit card debt, home mortgage, and property and income taxes.

You may want to arrange for the direct deposit into your savings or checking account of as many income sources as possible. To arrange for direct deposit of government funds (for example, Social Security and veterans' benefits), file an authorization form, which you can pick up at most banks.

A joint bank account in the names of both the person with Alzheimer's and the person who will be handling the finances is one way to simplify matters. However, there is a potential drawback. Although a joint account is a useful way to access another person's resources, it may cause complications if you apply for Medicaid or other benefits. Government programs assume that all money in a joint account belongs to the person applying for the benefit.

The durable power of attorney, described earlier, is probably the best option for turning over the management of financial affairs. The agent, who acts on behalf of the person with Alzheimer's disease, is authorized to deal with a wide range of financial matters, from managing bank accounts to selling assets.

To ease some of the financial burden, a few tax breaks exist for people with Alzheimer's and their caregivers. An accountant can help you figure out your eligibility. For example, you may be entitled to a tax credit for part of the cost of a home attendant. If you claim the person with Alzheimer's disease as a dependent, you may be able to deduct some medical expenses from your income tax.

Paying for health care

The costs of caring for a person with Alzheimer's disease are often high. There are some potential resources to help defray costs. These include Medicare, Medicaid, and private insurance.

Medicare

Medicare covers all people 65 and older who are receiving Social Security retirement benefits. It pays for hospital care, a portion of doctor's fees, some prescription drug costs, and some other medical expenses. For example, it covers physical and speech therapy and part of the cost of mental health care.

For dementia patients, Medicare will pay for physical, occupational, and speech therapy if the patient's doctor deems these services necessary. Medicare will also cover psychotherapy or behavior management therapy provided by a mental health professional if this type of therapy is deemed to be reasonable and helpful.

Medicare does not cover adult day care, 24-hour personal care in the home, or room and board in an assisted-living facility or nursing home. The exception is care received after a hospital stay of three or more days. In this case, Medicare will pay for home care or care in a skilled nursing facility, but only for a limited time.

Medicare prescription drug coverage is provided by private insurance companies. Medicare beneficiaries must choose a plan and pay a monthly premium. All Medicare drug plans cover the costs for cholinesterase inhibitor drugs (Aricept, Exelon, Razadyne) and Namenda, in addition to antidepressants, antipsychotics, and anticonvulsants.

Medicaid

Medicaid will cover the cost of long-term care for a person with Alzheimer's disease who meets the requirements. The laws are different, depending on the state in which you live, but benefits can include adult day care, respite care, home care, hospital care, and nursing home care. However, because it is a welfare program, the person with Alzheimer's disease must have minimal income and assets to qualify. Some people divest themselves of their assets in order to qualify for Medicaid. If you choose to do this, there will be a period of time (up to three years) during which Medicaid will not pay for your nursing home care. Before divesting your assets, consult with an attorney or financial planner who understands the Medicaid laws in your state.

Other financial help

Veterans and their spouses, widows, children, or parents may be eligible for some medical benefits from the Department of Veterans Affairs. These benefits can include adult day care, home care, outpatient care, hospital care, and nursing home care. Contact the U.S. Department of Veterans Affairs (800-827-1000) for more information.

It's possible to purchase long-term care insurance (nursing home insurance) from many insurance companies. These policies differ, but many are set up to pay a predetermined amount of money for each day a person is cared for in a long-term care facility. There can be deductibles, waiting periods, benefit time limits, and exclusions. Review several different plans before selecting one, and read the policy carefully before signing up. You typically must purchase long-term care insurance in advance of a disability. Once a person is diagnosed with Alzheimer's, obtaining long-term care insurance is difficult, because the disease is considered a pre-existing condition, and the policy probably won't cover it.

THE FUTURE OF ALZHEIMER'S RESEARCH

Over the past several years, many promising new treatments for Alzheimer's disease have emerged from research laboratories and raised hope initially, only to be found lacking when subjected to more rigorous study. But trial and error is the nature of medical advancement. Through this process, researchers believe they are getting closer to unraveling the mysteries of the multi-faceted puzzle of Alzheimer's disease. As fresh knowledge is gained, new ways of approaching the illness have emerged.

Researchers now pin their hopes for preventing or slowing Alzheimer's disease on developing treatments that can be given to people before any symptoms are noticeable. Therefore, research is focused on detecting the earliest changes in the brains of people with Alzheimer's disease and finding therapies to halt the progression. The focus has shifted from trying to cure people who already have symptoms of the disease to predicting who will get it and trying to stop it before irreversible damage to the brain sets in.

The biological changes in the brain may begin 15 to 20 years before diminished memory or other mental dysfunction is noticeable. Therefore, it is widely believed that the best hope for treating Alzheimer's disease will involve a therapy or combination of therapies taken in the very earliest stage of the disease—before symptoms arise. Breakthroughs in at least two areas must occur for this to become a reality. First, diagnostic tests must be developed that can accurately predict which healthy-appearing people or people with mild memory problems are actually in the early stage of Alzheimer's disease. Second, drugs or other therapies must be developed that can be used at that early stage to stop the illness.

Advancements are occurring on both fronts. New tests are being created that detect the earliest changes.

Drugs being developed are intended to alter the course of the disease itself. Several drugs with this disease-modifying effect have not been shown to be useful when given to people who already have the memory and thinking impairments of Alzheimer's disease. Many experts believe this is because they must be given in the very early stage before any problems with memory or thinking occur. Consequently, several studies are looking at giving drugs to people who have no symptoms of dementia but have a genetic

BOX 11-1

Research studies—should you participate?

It generally takes many years for scientific discoveries to bring about treatments that can be used in everyday medical practice. People with Alzheimer's disease may want to consider volunteering for research studies in order to participate in this process. Even people without the disease may benefit from getting involved in research. Researchers often recruit people without Alzheimer's disease to serve as healthy control subjects, or to identify risk factors.

For people with Alzheimer's disease, participation in clinical studies has several advantages. For example, you may be given an experimental treatment, and even if you aren't helped by the treatment, you may get satisfaction from knowing that you have been involved in the process of finding better treatments for future Alzheimer's patients. Additionally, people involved in clinical studies are usually treated by experts in the field, and they have access to more comprehensive health care than they probably would have otherwise.

However, there are some potential drawbacks to participating in research studies. The researcher's primary goal is to learn something about the disease and to answer specific scientific questions. To do this, they often compare the treatment with an inactive placebo, which means that you may receive a placebo and not be aware of it. Anyone considering taking part in a research study should read the consent forms very carefully, discuss the pros and cons with his or her personal physician, and understand exactly what is expected.

HOW TO PARTICIPATE

For those interested in participating in research, the National Institute on Aging maintains the Alzheimer's Disease Clinical Trials Database (www.nia.nih.gov/alzheimers). This Internet database lists clinical trials on Alzheimer's disease and dementia that are being conducted at medical centers throughout the United States. If you don't own a computer with Internet access, visit your local library. Most libraries are hooked up to the Internet.

predisposition to the disease or test positive on tests showing they are at high risk.

The failure of the new drugs to produce a dramatic improvement also points to the likelihood that no single drug alone will do the trick. Researchers are starting to believe that the multifaceted nature of Alzheimer's disease will require a combination of treatments.

Drug approval

Before a new drug is approved by the Food and Drug Administration it must pass through three phases of clinical trials. In Phase 1, the drug is tested in a small number of people to evaluate its safety and identify side effects. In Phase 2 trials, the treatment is given to a larger group of people to see if it works as intended. If those studies show effectiveness, the drug moves on to Phase 3, where it is tested in even larger groups of people to confirm the benefit and monitor side effects.

Many people with Alzheimer's disease and their families choose to participate in clinical trials. There are several advantages to such participation. For example, the treatment being studied may prove effective, and you will have access to it before it becomes publicly available. See Box 11-1, "Research studies—should you participate?" for a discussion of some issues to consider before participating in a clinical trial. For information on clinical trials in your area, check the websites listed in *Resources*, on page 96.

New methods of diagnosis

Today, the diagnosis of Alzheimer's disease is based on symptoms, medical history, and laboratory tests. But research is underway to develop diagnostic methods that more accurately make a positive diagnosis, and do so earlier in the course of the disease. Most of the imaging and other biomarkers discussed below are not ready for routine use in clinical practice, but they represent exciting possibilities for the future.

Because Alzheimer's disease begins to attack the brain years before the symptoms become apparent, many researchers are focused on finding "biomarkers" of Alzheimer's disease. A biomarker is something that can be measured in the body that indicates the presence or absence of a disease or the risk of later developing a disease. For example, cholesterol is a biomarker for heart disease. High cholesterol by itself does not cause symptoms, and people with high cholesterol do not know they have high cholesterol unless they have a blood test. But cholesterol is important because having high levels increases the risk for a stroke, heart attack, and other types of heart disease.

Researchers are looking for this kind of biomarker for Alzheimer's disease. For example, certain findings on new brain imaging techniques may serve as biomarkers. Researchers are also looking for proteins, genes, and other material present in either blood or cerebrospinal fluid (the fluid that bathes the brain and spine) that would signal the presence of the disease.

Brain imaging tests that can detect beta-amyloid or tau in the brain and tests of cerebrospinal fluid that show that beta-amyloid is present are already available. These tests can be invasive and/or expensive. They would be impractical to administer to large numbers of healthy-appearing people as screening tests to pick out those with very early Alzheimer's disease. Therefore, there also is a push to find initial screening tests that cost less and are easier to perform to narrow down those individuals who should receive the more advanced and complex tests. Ultimately, a combination of several types of tests will most likely be needed to identify people at the earliest stage of Alzheimer's disease.

Brain imaging studies

There are several ways to scan the brain to obtain an image. Positron emission tomography (PET) traces blood flow and metabolism (energy usage) in the brain. Magnetic resonance imaging (MRI) allows physicians to view a cross section of the brain and to measure the size of various brain structures. A type of MRI called functional MRI (fMRI) allows the physician to observe cross sections of the brain (and to see which areas are active) while the person is engaging in a mental activity, such as memorizing a list of words, speaking, or reading.

Scanning for plaques and tangles

Over the past several years, researchers have developed techniques that can create a direct picture of plaques and tangles in the living brain. These are called molecular imaging technologies. Just a few years ago, the only way to confirm the presence of plaques and tangles was to perform an autopsy after the person had died. But this is changing. One imaging method uses a compound that sticks to amyloid plaques (the brain abnormalities that indicate the presence of Alzheimer's disease) in the brain. This allows the clumps of amyloid to be visible with PET imaging.

Three compounds with the ability to stick to amyloid plaques have been approved by the FDA— florbetapir (Amyvid), flutemetamol F18 (Vizamyl), and florbetaben F18 (Neuraceq). Because these compounds have been approved for use by the FDA, they can be used by physicians to perform amyloid PET brain scans outside of a research setting. However, there are important limitations regarding the usefulness of this type of scan in general practice.

If the scan shows there are no amyloid plaques, then Alzheimer's disease is probably not the cause of any symptoms of dementia. Other causes should be considered. If plaques are detected, an Alzheimer's diagnosis would be possible. However, plaques can be present in the brains of people who don't have Alzheimer's disease, so other tests are needed to interpret the results of the scan.

The test has not been approved as a method to test people with normal mental function to determine if they will develop Alzheimer's disease, although this may happen in the future. In addition, special expertise is required to interpret the scan, which may cost about $2,500 to $3,000 and is not currently covered by private insurance or Medicare. A PET scan using molecular imaging technology may be most useful for differentiating different types of dementia.

Another type of PET study detects the presence of tau, which is the other substance in the brain that distinguishes Alzheimer's disease. This abnormal protein is responsible for the neurofibrillary tangles (described in Chapter 1) in the brains of people with Alzheimer's disease. Several compounds that can detect tau have been developed and are being tested.

PET scans

PET imaging, without the compounds that bind to amyloid plaques or tau, is a potentially reliable method for distinguishing between different forms of dementia. For example, it may be useful for determining whether a person has Alzheimer's disease, dementia with Lewy bodies, or frontotemporal dementia. Currently, the Centers for Medicare and Medicaid Services (CMS), the agency that oversees Medicare, will pay for PET scans, but only when doctors are unclear as to whether a patient has Alzheimer's disease or the form of dementia called frontotemporal dementia.

MRIs

Studies with MRI—which provides a picture of the brain—have shown that this technology might be useful for early diagnosis. It appears that certain brain structures (the hippocampus and entorhinal cortex) are smaller than normal, even in the very early stages of Alzheimer's disease. MRI can also detect thinning in the brain's cerebral cortex. The cerebral cortex is a thin layer of tissue that covers the part of the brain called the cerebrum. It plays a key role in memory, attention, thought and language. One study found that people who were cognitively normal and found to have thinning of the cerebral cortex were at greater risk for developing Alzheimer's disease.

A modified version of an MRI called arterial spin labeling (ASL-MRI) is being studied as a possible method to diagnose early dementia. This test is similar to an MRI, with the additional ability to look for changes in blood flow and the uptake of glucose (sugar) in the parts of the brain involved with memory. These changes can indicate altered brain function that may signal a person has dementia.

Cerebrospinal fluid markers

Some studies have indicated that the key biomarker may lie in cerebrospinal fluid. Cerebrospinal fluid is a clear liquid that bathes the brain and spinal cord. The brain continuously produces cerebrospinal fluid, which is then reabsorbed.

People with Alzheimer's disease appear to have reduced levels of a type of beta-amyloid called beta-amyloid 42, as well as increased levels of tau in their cerebrospinal fluid. Therefore, it has been hypothesized that measuring levels of these substances in healthy older adults might be used to predict who will later develop Alzheimer's disease.

Studies have shown that measuring levels of three proteins (total tau protein, phosphorylated tau, and beta-amyloid 42) in cerebrospinal fluid could predict which study participants would develop Alzheimer's disease. One study found that the presence of a protein called soluble amyloid precursor protein beta in cerebrospinal fluid may also be predictive.

One drawback of this type of testing is the need to perform a spinal tap (also called a lumbar puncture) to collect a sample of cerebrospinal fluid for testing. A spinal tap involves inserting a needle into the spinal canal in the lower back to draw out cerebrospinal fluid.

Neuropsychological tests

Neuropsychological tests, done even 10 years before the appearance of Alzheimer's symptoms, may offer clues to early warning signs.

In a study from Sweden, researchers combined the results from 47 different studies and found some specific changes in memory and cognition that, although subtle, are more common in people who

BOX 11-2

BETA-AMYLOID FORMATION

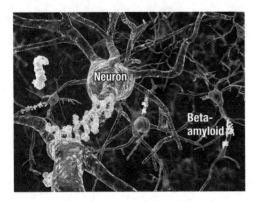

APP is a normal protein that aids in the health of neurons in the brain. It is broken down into shorter pieces by several groups of enzymes called secretases. One of these pieces is beta-amyloid, which can build up in the brain to form toxic plaque.

later develop Alzheimer's disease than in people who do not. The changes in cognition for people who later developed Alzheimer's disease were not that pronounced at first and did not differ greatly from some of the normal changes in memory that can occur in people who don't develop the disease. But a comprehensive battery of neuropsychological tests could detect the difference between normal changes and changes that indicate Alzheimer's disease.

Blood and other tests

An especially sought-after screening for early detection would be a blood test. Ideally, a simple blood test could be used to indicate whether a person is at greater-than-normal risk for Alzheimer's disease. This could then be followed up with more advanced types of screening tests. Many attempts have been made to develop such a blood test. Several groups of researchers have found different proteins in the blood that might have this predictive ability. Tests for these proteins are not yet ready for routine use, but researchers hope that a blood test may be available in the near future.

Several studies found that changes in a person's gait (such as slowing of walking pace or variable stride) may be an early indication of a decline in cognitive function, which may signal Alzheimer's disease. If a physician observes changes in a patient's gait that cannot be explained by other causes, cognitive testing may be warranted.

Potential treatment approaches

Scientists know that the brains of people with Alzheimer's disease contain plaques and tangles (see Chapter 1). The accumulation of these substances in the brain causes brain cells to die. As more and more brain cells die, the characteristic memory and thinking problems of Alzheimer's disease become apparent. One approach to treating the disease is to figure out what causes this process to get started, understand the cascade of events that follows the initial event, and intervene early in the process to stop it.

According to one theory, accumulation of beta-amyloid in the brain is the trigger that sets off the chain of events that culminates in the disease. Beta-amyloid is the toxic protein that is the major component of the sticky plaques in the brains of people with Alzheimer's disease (see Box 11-2, "Beta-amyloid formation"). Starting in middle age, beta-amyloid starts to form in just about everyone's brain, but it accumulates to a much greater degree in the brains of people with Alzheimer's disease.

Some as-yet-unknown trigger causes excessive amounts of beta-amyloid to form. This sets in motion all of the other biological processes, such as the development of the tangles, oxidation, inflammation, and the eventual death of brain cells.

Some Alzheimer's researchers are not convinced that the accumulation of beta-amyloid into plaques is the singular event that sets off all of the other brain changes in the disease. They point to other possibilities. An unknown factor may trigger the formation of tangles, which then leads to the plaques and eventual cell death. Or an unknown factor could cause the formation of both tangles and plaques simultaneously. Or there may be two triggers, one that causes plaques and the other that causes tangles.

There are many other possibilities as well, relating to the complexities of brain function. The constellation of damaging processes in the brains of people with Alzheimer's disease (plaques, tangles, inflammation, oxidation, and others) provides several targets for intervening with potential treatments to protect the brain.

Anti-amyloid approaches

If the accumulation of beta-amyloid is the initial trigger for the brain changes in Alzheimer's disease, then preventing beta-amyloid from forming in the brain or clearing the beta-amyloid already there would, theoretically, prevent or halt the disease. Many drugs and other therapies based on the beta-amyloid theory have been developed and are being tested. Some work by preventing beta-amyloid from forming, and others work by removing beta-amyloid that's already there.

Clearing beta-amyloid from the brain

One approach to clearing beta-amyloid from the brain harnesses the capability of the body's natural defenses to eliminate it. The immune system recognizes excess beta-amyloid as a threat and makes antibodies against it. Antibodies launch attacks against detrimental substances in the body. Boosting the levels of anti-amyloid antibodies has shown some promise.

Scientists have singled out the antibody against beta-amyloid and turned it into a drug therapy. Several such drugs have been developed, including solanezumab, crenezumab, and aducanumab, which bind to beta-amyloid and clear it away. These drugs showed promise in early studies with small numbers of patients. But when tested in large studies of people with mild-to-moderate Alzheimer's disease the results were disappointing.

Experimental Alzheimer's drug shows promise

When tested in two large phase 3 clinical trials, the drug solanezumab did not work for people with mild-to-moderate Alzheimer's disease. But it did seem to slow mental decline when the researchers looked only at those in the mild stage.

To further test the drug, the researchers extended the two 18-month studies, offering all participants the option to take the drug. This means that those who originally were in the group receiving a placebo (an inactive substance used to compare the active drug against) could now take the drug. These people would be starting the drug 18 months later than those originally in the group receiving the drug.

Comparing these two groups those—who had been taking the drug from the beginning of the study and those who started it 18 months later—could indicate whether the treatment actually slows the worsening of the condition. If the treatment actually slows down the disease, both groups would benefit but those who started it later would not be able to catch up in terms of mental function with those who started it earlier. That is what was found in this study in the participants with mild Alzheimer's disease, suggesting that solanezumab may have a disease-modifying effect.

Alzheimer's Association International Conference, July 2015

But the story does not end there. The drug solanezumab failed to improve mental function in people with mild-to-moderate Alzheimer's disease in two phase 3 studies that lasted 18 months. But, when researchers looked only at those in the mild stage they saw a glimmer of hope. The drug did slow mental decline. It is now being studied in a larger number of people with mild Alzheimer's disease. The results of that study are expected in 2017. In the meantime, the researchers extended the two phase 3 trials, offering all participants the option of taking the drug. The results of this study, which was presented at the 2015 Alzheimer's Association International Conference, showed that the drug might actually be promising (see Box 11-3 "Experimental Alzheimer's drug shows promise").

Crenezumab is also being studied in people with mild Alzheimer's disease.

Several experts believe that to be effective, these drugs must be given even earlier in the course of the disease, possibly before any symptoms are apparent. Studies in people at high risk for Alzheimer's disease but who do not yet have symptoms are underway (see "Studies in very early-stage Alzheimer's disease," page 89).

Prevent beta-amyloid from forming

Getting rid of beta-amyloid that's already formed in the brain is one option. Another strategy is to prevent the beta-amyloid from forming in the first place. As stated earlier, beta-amyloid is created from a larger protein called amyloid precursor protein (APP). APP is a normal protein that aids in the growth and maintenance of brain cells. The long strand of APP can be cut into smaller fragments. An enzyme acts like a pair of scissors cutting a long ribbon into shorter pieces. One of those pieces is beta-amyloid.

Scientists have identified the two enzymes that clip APP at just the right places to create beta-amyloid. They are called beta-secretase and gamma-secretase. Researchers have also identified another enzyme called alpha-secretase. This one is important because it snips the APP right in the middle of the region where beta-amyloid would be. This makes it impossible for beta-amyloid to form.

These findings are important because a drug that blocks the snipping action of beta-secretase or gamma-secretase would prevent beta-amyloid from forming. Conversely, a drug that boosts the production of alpha-secretase could have the same effect.

Several drugs that block either beta-secretase or gamma-secretase are being studied. One of them is a drug called verubecestat (made by Merck), which blocks beta-secretase. Early studies of this drug showed that it reduces levels of beta-amyloid in cerebrospinal fluid. Study participants who received the drug had lower levels of beta-amyloid than those receiving placebo. Larger phase 3 studies of this drug are underway.

The future for these types of drugs is uncertain. A potential drawback of drugs that block the action of the molecular scissors gamma- and beta-secretase is that these enzymes may have other, beneficial purposes. Also, not all beta-amyloid is harmful. Scientists have found that there are different types of beta-amyloid, some of which may be beneficial. Therefore, if the action of the snipping enzymes (gamma- and beta-secretase) is blocked completely, there might be unwanted side effects.

Studies in very early-stage Alzheimer's disease

Based on the belief that treatment for Alzheimer's disease must be given very early, several studies are underway to test this theory and to find the right drug for effective early intervention.

One study is using the drug crenezumab in people who have the gene that guarantees they will get Alzheimer's disease but do not yet have any symptoms. Only about one percent of people with Alzheimer's disease have this genetically determined form of the disease, but the results from this study may apply to the more common form of the disease. The researchers are hoping to show that by giving a drug to people who are cognitively normal now but are sure to get the disease later, it may be possible to prevent it from happening or at least to delay the onset.

The 300 participants in the study come from an extended family in Colombia, South America, and many of them carry a genetic mutation that results in dementia by age 51. Participants will receive either crenezumab or placebo, and will undergo several tests of cognitive functioning and other biomarkers of Alzheimer's disease. The study is expected to be completed in 2017.

DIAN TU

Another study is being conducted by the Dominantly Inherited Alzheimer's Network Trials Unit (DIAN TU) at Washington University School of Medicine. The participants in this study also carry the gene for genetically-determined Alzheimer's disease. This study is testing three different drugs. One is solanezumab (described earlier). The other two include another antibody drug called gantenerumab, which removes beta-amyloid plaques from the brain, and a drug that blocks the action of beta-secretase, thus preventing beta-amyloid from forming.

A4

The National Institutes of Health is funding a study called the Anti-Amyloid Treatment in Asymptomatic Alzheimer's disease (nicknamed A4). The participants in this study are not carriers of the genes for genetically determined Alzheimer's disease. Instead, the 1,000 participants are adults age 70 to 85 without obvious impairments in mental function as measured on tests of memory and thinking but who have evidence of buildup of beta-amyloid plaques in the brain as measured on amyloid PET scans. This suggests that they may develop dementia. The study, which will last three years, is testing whether solanezumab prevents or delays the onset of Alzheimer's disease.

Targeting tau and tangles

Many researchers are focusing their attention on neurofibrillary tangles. The tangles are caused by a protein called tau that has undergone detrimental changes. Cells use tau to construct microscopic tubes (microtubules) that allow movement of communication signals throughout the cell. In people with Alzheimer's disease, the tau becomes misshapen and turns into disorderly twisted fibers called tangles. When this happens, the cell loses its ability to communicate with other cells, and has more difficulty taking care of and repairing itself.

Scientists are investigating the exact role of tau and tangles in the development of Alzheimer's disease, as well as possible therapies to repair or prevent the tangles.

Tangles cause microtubules to become unstable. Some research aims to prevent this. In addition, it has been discovered that abnormal tau can spread from one neuron to neighboring neurons, thus causing a chain reaction that destroys millions of neurons. One line of research focuses on blocking this process.

Inhaled insulin

Another approach to treating Alzheimer's disease involves the relationship between insulin and brain function. Insulin, which is produced in the pancreas, transports glucose (sugar) into cells, where it is used as a source of energy. Levels of insulin and glucose must be maintained at the proper balance for optimal function of cells, including brain cells. When the body does not produce enough insulin or does not properly use it, the result is diabetes.

Type 2 diabetes is caused by insulin resistance, which means the body no longer responds sufficiently to the effects of insulin. Insulin resistance starts slowly and worsens over time until a threshold level is reached, at which point diabetes is diagnosed. Insulin resistance itself (even before it becomes diabetes) can have detrimental effects. Over time, insulin resistance can cause increased inflammation and the accumulation of beta-amyloid in the brain. People with Alzheimer's disease may have insulin resistance.

Given this possible connection, researchers hypothesized that delivering insulin to the brain may have a beneficial effect. In a small study, a group of researchers tested whether inhaled insulin would slow the progression of Alzheimer's disease. In the study older adults with mild cognitive impairment or mild-to-moderate Alzheimer's disease received insulin in the form of a nasal spray or placebo for four months. Treatment with a lower dose of insulin (20 international units [IU]) improved memory, and treatment with a low (20 IU) or higher (40 IU) dose preserved general cognition and functional ability. Based on the positive findings from this study, the National Institutes of Health has funded a larger study, which is underway.

Other approaches

Researchers are attacking the disease from many other angles in addition to those discussed above. Some scientists have come up with new theories about the cause of Alzheimer's disease. While the amyloid hypothesis and research on tau have received much of the focus, there may be other substances in the brain worth examining. For example, a group of researchers believes that beta-amyloid oligomers are to blame rather than beta-amyloid plaques. Oligomers are floating clumps of beta-amyloid. The researchers created a genetically modified mouse that forms only oligomers and never plaques. In a study, these mice were just as cognitively impaired as their counterparts that develop plaques and oligomers.

Researchers are also looking into ways to protect brain cells and reduce inflammation in the brain.

Stem cell research

Curing diseases by replacing failing body systems with regenerated cells is perhaps the "Holy Grail" of scientific research. This could be possible through stem cell research. Alzheimer's disease is just one of many conditions thought to potentially benefit from this approach. If it fulfills its promise, stem cell therapy could be used to create fresh nerve cells that would replace the ones depleted by Alzheimer's disease.

At this point in time, the potential of stem cell research exists (early experiments have shown it to be possible for at least some diseases), but the reality of translating research into actual treatments or cures is still a long way off. Specifically, stem cell research must overcome significant hurdles.

Put simply, stem cell research is based on the fact that some cells have the flexibility to become many different types of cells. The cells of the human body are mostly quite specialized. For example, there are skin cells, liver cells, blood cells and nerve cells. Stem cells are a type of cell with the potential to become any other type of cell.

The most versatile stem cells are embryonic stem cells. Bone marrow, which is the source of many kinds of blood cells, also contains stem cells. Stem cells can also be obtained from umbilical cords. Scientists discovered that they could stimulate stem cells to become specific types of cells. This breakthrough has led to ongoing research to see if it's possible to, for example, create insulin-producing cells for diabetics or nerve cells to replace faulty ones in the brains of people with Parkinson's disease.

The techniques for coaxing cells into becoming a desired type are far from perfected, and there are many factors that would need to be considered in relation to Alzheimer's, such as which types of cells would be replicated, which specific areas of the brain would be targeted, and how to get the cells to make the complicated connections found in the brain. And scientists still have to work out how they would introduce the new cells into patients and how they would ensure that the cells don't transform into an undesirable cell type—a cancer cell, for example.

Conclusion

Research is happening at many levels, from basic research conducted in laboratories in petri dishes to new drugs and therapies being tested in humans. Scientists are simultaneously figuring out how the disease starts and progresses, how to test for it, how to treat it, and how to prevent it. Different researchers are coming at the problem from different angles. Some day soon, one or more of these approaches may open the door to a world where Alzheimer's disease is on the decline.

Acetylcholine: A neurotransmitter in the parts of the brain involved in thinking, learning, and memory. (Neurotransmitters are chemicals that allow cells in the brain to communicate with one another.)

Adult day care: Adult day centers are facilities in which people with Alzheimer's and other dementias can be social and participate in activities in a safe environment.

Advanced directive: A legal document outlining what kind of medical treatment a person would like when he or she can no longer communicate such wishes.

Aggression: Acting in a manner that can harm oneself or other people.

Agitation: Emotional disturbance.

Allele: The basic biological makeup of living things (including humans) is guided by genes. Each gene codes for a particular trait or function. Variations of individual genes are called alleles. For example, having one allele will code for black hair, while having a different allele will code for blond hair.

Alzheimer's disease: The most common form of dementia. Memory, thinking, and behavior become progressively worse until a person requires help with most aspects of daily functioning.

Amyloid plaque: In the brains of people with Alzheimer's disease, protein pieces called beta-amyloid clump together to form a material called amyloid plaque. This impairs the ability of brain cells to function properly.

Amyloid precursor protein (APP): The beta-amyloid that clumps together to form amyloid plaques is a small piece of this larger protein.

Antibodies: These components of the immune system attack harmful substances in the body.

Anxiety: This response to stress causes feelings such as nervousness, fear, or apprehension. It can range from mild and unsettling to debilitating.

Aphasia: This is the term for difficulty speaking or understanding language, as well as difficulty reading and writing. It is caused by damage to certain areas of the brain and can occur in people in the later stages of Alzheimer's disease.

Apolipoprotein E (ApoE): A gene that provides instructions for making a protein that is also called apolipoprotein E. The protein is involved in the breakdown of fats in the body. People who carry an allele of the ApoE gene called ApoE4 are at increased risk for Alzheimer's disease.

Autopsy: A procedure performed on a body after death to determine the cause of death.

Behavior: The actions and reactions of a person in response to other people and to other aspects of their environment.

Beta-amyloid: Pieces of protein that can stick together to form amyloid plaques in the brains of people with Alzheimer's disease.

Biomarker: Something that can be measured in the body that indicates the presence or absence of disease or the risk for later developing a disease.

Cell: The basic building blocks of all living organisms. The human body has trillions of cells.

Cerebral cortex: The brain is composed of several parts. The cerebral cortex is the outermost layer, and it is responsible for higher brain functions, such as intelligence, personality, and planning and organizing.

Cerebrospinal fluid: The brain and spinal cord are surrounded by this clear fluid, which acts as a cushion.

Cholesterol: Cholesterol is a fat-like substance found in all cells of the body. It is necessary for certain normal functions of the body. However, excess amounts of a type of cholesterol called low-density lipoprotein (LDL) cholesterol can build up inside blood vessels, which can increase risk for heart disease and possibly Alzheimer's disease.

Cholinesterase inhibitors: These Alzheimer's disease drugs act on a neurotransmitter (chemicals that facilitate communication between brain cells) called acetylcholine. Acetylcholine is diminished in people with Alzheimer's disease. Cholinesterase inhibitor drugs (such as donepezil, rivastigmine, and galantamine) stop cholinesterase from deactivating acetylcholine, thus allowing more acetylcholine to remain in the brain.

Chromosome: The genetic code (DNA) is contained in each cell of the body. The genes are arranged on thread-like structures called chromosomes. In humans there are 23 pairs of chromosomes, for a total of 46.

CT scan (computed tomography): This diagnostic test uses x-ray beams to create a series of images of an internal body area. When put together the images provide a three-dimensional view of the area. People suspected of having dementia may have a CT scan of the brain to look for possible alternative causes of symptoms, such as a tumor or stroke.

Cognition: This refers to mental functions such as memory, orientation, language, judgment, and problem solving.

Daily plan: A schedule of activities that provide a person with Alzheimer's meaning and enjoyment, as well as a familiar structure that helps ease anxiety.

Dementia: A progressive illness that results in memory loss and other cognitive abnormalities that over time seriously interfere with daily life. There are several forms of dementia, the most common of which is Alzheimer's disease.

Depression: This mental illness is characterized by profound sadness that persists and adversely affects daily life.

Diabetes: People with this condition do not properly process glucose (from food that is eaten). This is because they either do not produce the hormone insulin (which is needed to transport glucose to cells, where it is converted into energy) or the body is unable to effectively use the insulin that is produced. People with diabetes are at increased risk for Alzheimer's disease.

DNA (deoxyribonucleic acid): This is the hereditary material inside of cells. Genes are composed of DNA.

Down syndrome: A condition that causes intellectual disability, a characteristic facial appearance, and weak muscle tone. Down syndrome is caused by a having an extra copy of chromosome 21. People with Down syndrome have an increased risk for developing several medical conditions, including Alzheimer's disease.

Entorhinal cortex: This brain structure is involved with memory. It is damaged in people with Alzheimer's disease.

Frontotemporal dementia: One of several forms of dementia. The frontal and temporal anterior lobes of the brain shrink, which leads to either changes in behavior or problems with language.

Gene: Genes code for physical traits like eye and hair color as well as many other functions of living organisms. Genes are made up of DNA. Each chromosome inside the nucleus (center) of a cell contains many genes. These are the basic units of heredity.

Glucose: A sugar used by the body as a source of energy. Food that is eaten is broken down in the digestive system into glucose.

Hallucination: Seeing, hearing, smelling or feeling something that doesn't exist.

Hippocampus: This brain structure plays an important role in memory. In people with Alzheimer's disease the hippocampus shrinks considerably.

Huntington's disease: This brain disorder causes uncontrolled movements, emotional problems, and cognitive impairment. It occurs in people who have a mutation (change) in a particular gene.

Immune system: The immune system is a complex system that defends the body against attacks by foreign invaders. It can recognize potentially dangerous substances (such as bacteria and viruses) and mount attacks via specialized cells.

Inflammation: When tissues of the body are injured by trauma, bacteria, heat, or other causes, inflammation (swelling) occurs. This is a response of the immune system that helps with getting rid of foreign substances and with healing. Sometimes inflammation persists beyond the time when it is useful and it can become harmful.

Lewy body dementia: One of several forms of dementia. Lewy bodies are microscopic proteins that can accumulate in the brain and cause mental decline. People with this type of dementia also have other symptoms, such as drowsiness, lethargy, visual hallucinations, physical rigidity, and loss of spontaneous movement.

MRI (magnetic resonance imaging): This diagnostic test uses a powerful magnet and radio waves to produce an image of an internal body area. An MRI of the brain may be performed in people with suspected dementia.

Microtubules: Microscopic tubes that allow movement of communication signals throughout cells.

Mild cognitive impairment: Problems with memory, language and other mental functions that are more pronounced than normal age-related changes but don't fulfill the criteria for dementia.

Mini-Mental State Examination (MMSE): A short test that measures a person's basic cognitive health, including short-term memory, long-term memory, writing and speaking.

Neurofibrillary tangles: Dense proteins within nerve cells in the brain that injure the cells. The tangles are twisted threads, the major component of which is a protein called tau. Along with amyloid plaques, this is a hallmark feature of Alzheimer's disease.

Neurons (also called nerve cells): There are numerous types of cells in the human body. The brain and spinal cord are composed of nerve cells. This type of cell has a cell body, several short branches (dendrites), and one long branch (axon). Nerve cells send signals (via neurotransmitters) down the axon, which are picked up by connecting cells at the dendrites.

Neurotransmitter: These are chemicals that allow cells in the brain to communicate with one another.

Palliative care: Medical care to ease the pain and help improve the quality of life for someone with a serious or terminal illness.

Parkinson's disease: In people with this disease brain cells that produce a neurotransmitter called dopamine are diminished. Dopamine-producing cells are essential for movement. People with Parkinson's disease have trembling hands, arms, legs, and face. They also have stiffness in the limbs, slow movement, and impaired balance and coordination. Some people with Parkinson's disease develop dementia.

PET scan (positron emission tomography): With this diagnostic test a small amount of a radioactive substance is infused into a vein. A scan is then performed that detects signals from the radioactive substance and produces a three-dimensional image of internal body structures.

Placebo: An inactive substance used in scientific studies of new drugs. In these studies, one group of patients will receive the drug being tested and a second group will receive the placebo. By comparing the two groups scientists can determine if the drug being tested worked.

Power of attorney: A legal form that names another person to make legal, financial and other decisions for someone who can no longer handle those responsibilities because of Alzheimer's or other compromising conditions.

Presenilins: Mutations of the two genes presenilin 1 and presenilin 2 are linked to early-onset Alzheimer's disease.

Respite care: Temporary relief from caregiving responsibilities. Examples include adult day care, in-home assistance and short nursing home stays.

Stages: The framework for describing the progression of Alzheimer's disease.

Wandering: An individual with Alzheimer's or other form of dementia is at risk of wandering away from his or her residence and becoming disoriented and lost, even in familiar surroundings.

Younger-onset Alzheimer's: When someone under the age of 65 develops Alzheimer's, the person is said to have younger-onset Alzheimer's.

For additional information on Alzheimer's disease, contact the following organizations:

Administration on Aging
202-619-0724
www.aoa.gov

Alzheimer's Association
225 North Michigan Avenue
Chicago, IL 60611-7633
800-272-3900 (24/7 helpline)
312-335-8700
www.alz.org/www.alzconnected.org

**Alzheimer's Disease Education
& Referral Center**
PO Box 8250
Silver Spring, MD 20907-8250
800-438-4380
www.nia.nih.gov/Alzheimers/

Care2Caregivers
151 Centennial Avenue
Piscataway, NJ 08854
800-424-2494
www.care2caregivers.com

**Alzheimer's Foundation
of America**
322 Eighth Avenue, 7th floor
New York, NY 10001
866-232-8484
www.alzfdn.org

**American Federation
for Aging Research**
55 West 39th Street, 16th Floor
New York, NY 10018
888-582-2327 or 212-703-9977
www.afar.org

**American Health
Assistance Foundation**
22512 Gateway Center Drive
Clarksburg, MD 20871
800-437-2423
www.ahaf.org

American Health Care Association
1201 L St. N.W.
Washington, D.C. 20005
202-842-4444
www.ahca.org

Eldercare Locator
800-677-1116
www.eldercare.gov

A non-profit federation of nursing home providers:

**Assisted Living Federation
of America**
1650 King St., Suite 602
Alexandria, VA 22317-2747
703-894-1805
www.alfa.org

Children of Aging Parents
P.O. Box 167
Richboro, PA, 18954-0167
800-227-7294
www.caps4caregivers.org

ElderLawAnswers
535 Boylston St., 8th Floor
Boston, MA 02116-3720
866-267-0947
www.ElderLawAnswers.com

**Center for Applied Research in
Dementia**
34194 Aurora Road, #182
Solon, OH 44139
330-631-9949
www.cen4ard.com

**National Association for
Home Care & Hospice**
228 Seventh Street, SE
Washington, DC 20003
202-547-7424
www.nahc.org

**National Association of
Professional Geriatric
Care Managers**
3275 West Ina Road, Suite 130
Tucson, AZ 85741-2198
520-881-8008
www.caremanager.org

**National Family
Caregivers Association**
10400 Connecticut Ave, Suite 500
Kensington, MD 20895-3944
800-896-3650
www.nfcacares.org

**National Hospice &
Palliative Care Organization**
1700 Diagonal Road, Suite 625
Alexandria, VA 22314
800-658-8898, 703-837-1500
www.nhpco.org

National Institutes of Health
www.alzheimers.gov

U.S. Department of Veterans Affairs
800-827-1000
www.va.gov